BSAVA Manual of Canine and Feline Wound Management and Reconstruction

Editors:

David Fowler

DVM MVSc Diplomate ACVS
Department of Veterinary Anesthesiology, Radiology & Surgery,
Western College of Veterinary Medicine, University of Saskatchewan,
Saskatoon, Saskatchewan, S7N 5B4, Canada

and

John M. Williams

MA VetMB CertVR FRCVS Diplomate ECVS
Oakwood Referrals, 267 Chester Road,
Hartford Road, Northwich, Cheshire CW8 1LP

appropriate literature.

Typeset by: Fusion Design, Fordingbridge, Hampshire, UK

Printed by: Lookers, Upton, Poole, Dorset

Other titles in the BSAVA Manuals series:

Contents

Contributors

Stephen J. Baines
MA VetMB CertVR CertSAS MRCVS
Department of Clinical Veterinary Medicine, University of Cambridge, Madingley Road, Cambridge CB3 0ES

Jamie R. Bellah
DVM Diplomate ACVS
University of Florida, College of Veterinary Medicine, Box 100126 HSC, Gainesville, FL 32610-0126, USA

Jonathan Chambers
DVM Diplomate ACVS
Department of Small Animal Medicine, University of Georgia, Athens, GA 30602, USA

David Fowler
DVM MVSc Diplomate ACVS
Department of Veterinary Anesthesiology, Radiology & Surgery, Western College of Veterinary Medicine,
University of Saskatchewan, Saskatoon, Saskatchewan, S7N 5B4, Canada

Clare R. Gregory
DVM Diplomate ACVS
2112 Medical Science 1A, Veterinary Medical Surgery, University of California at Davis, Davis,
CA 95616, USA

Audrey Remedios
DVM MVSc Diplomate ACVS
Department of Veterinary Anesthesiology, Radiology & Surgery, Western College of Veterinary Medicine,
University of Saskatchewan, Saskatoon, Saskatchewan, S7N 5B4, Canada

Richard A.S. White
BVetMed PhD DSAS DVR FRCVS Diplomate ACVS Diplomate ECVS RCVS Specialist in Small
Animal Surgery
Department of Clinical Veterinary Medicine, University of Cambridge, Madingley Road, Cambridge CB3 0ES

John M. Williams
MA VetMB CertVR FRCVS Diplomate ECVS RCVS Specialist in Small Animal Surgery (Soft Tissue)
Oakwood Referrals, 267 Chester Road, Hartford Road, Northwich, Cheshire CW8 1LP

Foreword

The expectations of pet owners regarding corrective and reconstructive surgery have undoubtedly been raised by the ever-increasing number of medical and veterinary clinical documentary style programmes on television. Moreover, surgery of this nature presents both a challenge to the surgeon and visible rewards in the case of a successful outcome.

During the production of this Manual, the Editors have made every effort to ensure that the text is copiously illustrated with excellent colour photographs, and that the various surgical techniques are clearly explained. The sections on skin grafting and complications of wound healing will be of particular interest to any veterinary surgeon presented with patients following road traffic accidents and include comprehensive advice on the postoperative therapeutic management of such cases.

The title of this Manual might appear slightly forbidding, but a glance at the various chapters of the book will illustrate that it contains much useful advice for the general practitioner, not just the ambitious surgeon.

John F.R. Hird
BSAVA President 1998–99

Preface

In the last 20 years canine and feline wound management has advanced dramatically. This has been based on a better understanding of wound healing and its potential problems as well as development of reconstructive techniques which range from basic tension relieving procedures through to the use of microvascular techniques. The goal of wound reconstruction is always to return the traumatized patient to normal function as cosmetically as possible, though the final aesthetic appearance is of secondary importance.

This manual will help you understand how wounds heal and why they sometimes do not heal as well as we would like, and will help you in the management process. The chapters will take you through the decision making from the basic principles: whether to close the wound; choosing an appropriate wound dressing; through to wound closure techniques. A vast array of closure techniques are discussed, from the use of simple tension relieving techniques, dealing with fluid accumulation, axial pattern skin flaps to skin grafting. Consideration is also given to deeper wounds and using either muscle flaps or microvascular reconstructive techniques.

This is a truly transatlantic venture with contributions from acknowledged experts in their field from both the UK and North America. The editors would like to thank the authors for their time and excellent contributions. This book has been long in 'construction' and we are indebted to Marion Jowett for her patience and gentle cajoling as deadlines approached.

This is the ideal book when faced with your next degloving injury.

John Williams
Dave Fowler
June 1999

CHAPTER ONE

Wound Management and Reconstruction

John M. Williams and David Fowler

INTRODUCTION

Over the past two decades, wound management and reconstruction has become an increasingly exciting and demanding area of veterinary surgery. Our knowledge of the biology of wound healing and of the factors that contribute to abnormal wound healing has expanded greatly. Open wound management has been revolutionized by the development of 'new' wound dressing products that serve to optimize the wound healing environment (see Chapter 5). Historically, wounds in veterinary patients were allowed to heal by second intention, or were reconstructed using relatively simple procedures. Many more advanced reconstructive techniques have been described more recently. Axial pattern skin flaps (see Chapter 8), pedicled muscle flaps (see Chapter 10) and microvascular free tissue transfer (see Chapter 11) have expanded the armamentarium of the reconstructive surgeon. Knowledgeable application of these newer reconstructive techniques has facilitated more rapid and more functional recoveries, with fewer wound-related complications.

It is important to remember that no one reconstructive technique should be considered superior to any other. Rather, the specific advantages and disadvantages of each reconstructive technique must be understood and matched to the requirements of the wound. In many cases a combination of techniques may be required to effect a satisfactory reconstruction.

The veterinary surgeon must always remember that wound reconstruction following trauma or oncological resection may be an exciting surgical challenge, but it must ultimately be for the benefit of the patient and

not the surgeon. Amputation may be preferable to reconstruction when faced with excessively debilitating extremity wounds.

The choice of reconstructive techniques suitable to any given case is not black and white. Accomplished surgeons differ in opinion and approach. The process of evaluation and decision making is demonstrated in Chapter 14. Future prospective clinical research will undoubtedly lead to more specific recommendations, but it is important to realize that there will always be a great deal of latitude in the selection of reconstructive options, so long as the surgeon adheres to basic principles.

THE GOAL OF WOUND RECONSTRUCTION

The goal of wound reconstruction is to return the individual to the best possible function as quickly as possible and with the best cosmetic results. To achieve this goal, it is imperative that the veterinary surgeon understands the basic biology of wound healing, the reconstructive options available, factors that may affect the wound positively or negatively, and potential adverse sequelae. The art of successful wound reconstruction is to match management and reconstructive techniques optimally to the specific requirements of the wound.

BASIC SURGICAL PRINCIPLES

As with all surgery, wound reconstruction relies heavily on the basic principles of surgery which were put forward by Halstead in 1911 (Figure 1.1) and these should be closely adhered to. Performing surgery without regard to the surviving tissues will inevitably lead to failure.

Halstead's principles can be augmented by ensuring that tissues do not dry out under hot theatre lights and that correct instrumentation is used. Instruments used to handle delicate tissues, such as the skin, should cause minimal trauma. Coarse rat-toothed forceps and Allis tissue forceps have no role to play in reconstructive surgery. Skin edges should be handled as little as

Gentle tissue handling
Accurate haemostasis
Preservation of local blood supply
Aseptic technique
Close tissues without tension
Careful approximation of tissues
Ensure no dead space

Figure 1.1: Halstead's principles of surgery.

Type of injury	Time to act	Examples
Very severe/life-threatening injury	Must act within minutes	Cardiac arrest Airway obstruction Respiratory arrest Rapid arterial/venous haemorrhage
Severe	Must act within the first hour	Hypovolaemia Shock Penetrating wounds to thorax or abdomen Loss of consciousness Respiratory distress Spinal trauma and neurological deficits
Serious	Must act within the first few hours	Multiple deep lacerations Blunt trauma Moderate degree of shock Compound fractures Septicaemia
Major	Need to act within 24 hours	Fractures Deep puncture wounds

Figure 1.2: *Triage organization chart.*

possible and fine instruments such as skin hooks, Debakey or fine-toothed Adson forceps are least traumatic. Alternatively, fine monofilament stay sutures can be used. All incisions should be carried out with a scalpel and not scissors, as the latter crush and tear tissues. Similarly, sutures and suture material should be of fine gauge monofilament with swaged on reverse cutting needles used. Needle holders are often a matter of personal preference but should be fine tipped so as not to break and to allow accurate placement.

PATIENT EVALUATION

Initial evaluation of the trauma patient

When presented with a dog or cat which has been involved in trauma, resulting in a grotesque open wound, it is all too easy to concentrate on the wound and to forget that other body systems may also be traumatized. It is therefore essential on presentation to *evaluate fully* the injured patient to ensure that there are no other life-threatening injuries. Following initial evaluation it is equally essential to manage the whole patient appropriately.

It is vital to develop a routine for rapid but accurate evaluation of the trauma patient, which allows full assessment of vital parameters and the institution of rapid life-preserving measures when required. With all trauma patients the most important step is to determine that there is a patent airway and that the cardiorespiratory system is functional; all other body systems are secondary to this.

It is useful to use charts or plans to ensure that no systems are missed. Figure 1.2 outlines one such plan, which gives general guidelines as to which types of trauma must be dealt with immediately and which may be safely left. It is, however, important to realize that any injured patient may destabilize rapidly and therefore all patients should be assessed at regular intervals.

In addition to a broad sweep assessment it is useful to have an organized rapid system for evaluating the patient. An example is shown in Figure 1.3.

In evaluating a patient following trauma, consideration should be given, where appropriate, to radiography; this should not only cover the affected part of the body (e.g. the pelvis or a distal limb) but also include thoracic radiography to look for evidence of air or fluid within the thorax. Limb fractures will of necessity require management, and the surgeon must prioritize what needs to be dealt with first. The use of external fixators has helped considerably in the management of fractures associated with open wounds (see

A	Airway
C	Cardiovascular
R	Respiratory
A	Abdomen
S	Spine
H	Head
P	Pelvis
L	Limbs
A	Arteries
N	Nerves

Figure 1.3: *A CRASH PLAN.*

the *BSAVA Manual of Small Animal Fracture Repair and Management*). External fixators may be applied early following presentation, where other methods of fixation may be inappropriate, and will allow any open wound to be dressed as needed.

In the initial period it is important to remember that the traumatized patient will be suffering pain and that this must be attended to. The choice is that of the individual veterinary surgeon and will require judicious use of opioids and/or non-steroidal anti-inflammatory drugs (NSAIDs) as the situation dictates.

A full discussion on trauma management is outside the scope of this chapter and readers are referred to the *BSAVA Manual of Canine and Feline Emergency and Critical Care* and the reading list.

It is inevitable that in some situations, wound management and return to normal function may not be possible. For example, where there is a severe wound to a distal extremity the surgeon should consider the possibility of limb amputation or, in some extreme situations, euthanasia. It is essential not to lose sight of the fact that, despite advances in wound care and reconstruction, we must provide the patient with an adequate quality of life. In some cases it is also important to remember that not all clients can afford extensive and expensive management.

Evaluation of the cancer patient

Many major advances in reconstructive surgery have been in response to the development of aggressive veterinary oncological surgery. A greater understanding of the biology of tumours, in particular the sarcomas, has moved the surgeon away from simple 'lumpectomies' to radical excisions. Such deficits have meant that the surgeon must not only plan to excise a tumour with adequate margins but must also plan how to close the resultant wound.

In evaluating a patient with a solid tumour it is necessary to stage the patient according to the TNM classification system (Figure 1.4; Owen, 1980). Such staging allows the veterinary surgeon to gauge the full extent and type of the primary tumour, together with knowledge as to whether it has spread within the patient; such information is essential to arrive at an accurate prognosis and treatment strategy. The surgeon and the client must have the maximum amount of information possible so that an informed judgement can be made on management.

The minimum database available for an oncological case should be:

TNM STAGING SYSTEM	
T	Primary Tumour
N	Regional Lymph Nodes
M	Distant Metastasis

Figure 1.4: The TNM tumour classification system.

- Histology of the primary tumour (biopsies must be planned such that all biopsy tracts can be subsequently excised at time of surgical resection)
- Size and full extent of primary tumour
- Evaluation of local draining lymph nodes for metastatic spread
- Radiographic evaluation of the thorax for evidence of distant spread
- With certain tumour types, it may be necessary to assess other organs and body systems with radiography, ultrasonography, computerized tomography or magnetic resonance imaging.

Although surgery remains the cornerstone for the management of most solid tumours, it is essential to understand the roles of chemotherapy, radiotherapy and immunotherapy in designing an optimal treatment plan. The surgeon should work closely with medical oncologists, pathologists and radiologists so that appropriate multimodality treatment can be instituted. This may include pre- or postoperative chemotherapy, radiotherapy or immunotherapy. If such management is planned, it is essential that the timing of surgery is such that adjunctive therapy has the minimum deleterious effect on wound healing.

Planning management and reconstruction

All wounds are *not* created equal. The veterinary surgeon has an opportunity to control the wound environment in surgically created tissue deficits (e.g. tumour resections). Particular attention is paid to minimizing contamination, preserving vascular supply, and limiting tissue trauma. In contrast, the surgeon has no control over the initial status of traumatic wounds. A thorough understanding of the wound's aetiology, the degree of contamination, the likelihood of significant vascular disruption, and the potential for ongoing tissue necrosis is imperative. These factors are discussed in more detail in Chapter 4.

The depth of tissue injury and the involvement of 'critical' tissues or structures must also be considered. Traumatic wounds associated with long bone fracture (grade III b open fracture) or with exposed neurovascular structures benefit from early reconstruction using well vascularized tissues. Early reconstruction of the fracture using muscle flaps is associated with a lower incidence of osteomyelitis, an earlier onset of callus formation and more rapid union. Superficial wounds are amenable to more prolonged periods of open wound management, allowing delayed reconstruction or second intention healing.

Successful reconstruction of any wound relies on careful planning; it is probably best if the surgeon has more than one plan in mind. One of the leading human, plastic and reconstructive surgeons of the twentieth century, Sir Harold Gillies, was quoted as saying 'Never do today what can best be done tomorrow' (Converse, 1977). Although thorough preoperative planning should lead to identification of an optimal reconstructive strategy, occasionally we find that the initial reconstructive plan is inadequate due to poor local or distant blood supply or, in the case of oncological surgery, because the original excision becomes larger than was initially anticipated. The most successful reconstructions tend to be those where the surgeon had more than one plan in mind at the outset and was prepared to implement back-up strategies without further delay.

REFERENCES AND FURTHER READING

Converse JM (1977) *Reconstructive Plastic Surgery.* WB Saunders, Philadelphia

Coughlan A and Miller A (1998) *BSAVA Manual of Small Animal Fracture Repair and Management.* BSAVA, Cheltenham

King L and Hammond R (1999) *BSAVA Manual of Canine and Feline Emergency and Critical Care.* BSAVA, Cheltenham

Owen LN (1980) *TNM Classification of Tumours in Domestic Animals.* WHO, Geneva

CHAPTER TWO

The Aetiology and Classification of Wounds and Skin Deficits

Richard A.S. White

The treatment of wounds is a branch of the greatest importance in the practice of farriery yet it is very imperfectly understood, and many foolish and injurious opinions are entertained on the subject.

Lawson, *Modern Farrier*, 1832

INTRODUCTION

A wound can be defined as:

An interruption in the continuity of the external surface of the body or of the surface of an internal organ.

This chapter examines those aspects of the aetiology and classification of wounds that relate specifically to the external surface and its associated structures. Since wounds have a wide variety of aetiologies and their patterns of tissue trauma vary considerably, it follows that the clinician must have a thorough appreciation of their causation and complications in order to provide the most effective treatment for the individual wound type. Although initially the clinician's attention may be drawn to the superficial part of the wound or to the skin deficit itself, it is often the severity of bacterial

contamination within the wounded tissues and the associated trauma that determine patient morbidity. For that reason and despite the fact that there is no universally accepted wound classification system it is useful to categorize wounds according to their aetiology since this will usually provide some indication of their likely complications in terms of:

- The severity and complexity of the skin deficit
- The likely degree of accompanying bacterial contamination
- The extent of trauma to the surrounding tissues.

INCISIONAL INJURIES

Aetiology

Incisions are created by a sharp object moving in a plane parallel to the skin surface. The incising object is most commonly a scalpel blade at the beginning of a surgical procedure but in traumatic wounds it may be a glass fragment or a jagged tin edge responsible for the wound. Incisional wounds are typified by their clean, regular edges which gape open as the result of the inherent elasticity of the adjacent skin (Figures 2.1 and 2.2). Depending on its aetiology, the depth of the incision can vary considerably along its length and despite minimal involvement of the surrounding tissue

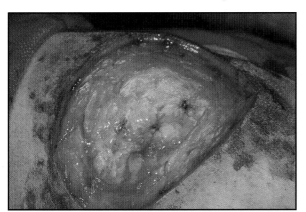

Figure 2.1: *Incisional wound. The clean surgically incised wound is characterized by regular edges, minimal trauma to the associated tissues and has little opportunity for contamination.*

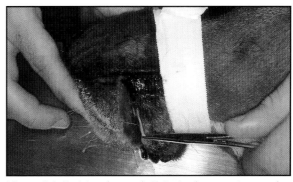

Figure 2.2: *Incisional wound. An incised traumatic wound resulting from the malicious placement of an elastic band over the lower jaw. Note that despite its traumatic aetiology the wound still retains regular, well defined edges with little damage apparent to the deeper tissues.*

there may be extension to the deeper tissues resulting in section of muscles, tendons or nerves.

Complications

The mechanism of the injury does not lend itself to inoculation of microorganisms into the wound and consequently incisions tend to be free of major contamination. Additionally, incised wounds bleed freely and this irrigating and cleansing effect is valuable in terms of preventing what superficial bacterial contamination there may be from becoming established in the tissues. Incisions are for the most part, therefore, much less prone to infection than other types of wounds and this often permits their safe primary closure at a comparatively early stage. The edges of the wound and surrounding tissues are rarely contused but exploration of the full depth of the wound is indicated to ensure that trauma to deeper structures is not overlooked.

ABRASIONS

Aetiology

An abrasion refers to damage caused to the epidermis and superficial dermis by frictional contact with a surface moving in a plane parallel to that of the skin. In practice, this term is also often used to refer to any wound caused through abrasive injury, even though tissues much deeper than the dermis may be involved. In small animal practice, abrasions are most commonly encountered in road traffic injuries and occur as the animal becomes trapped between the road surface and the moving vehicle with either, or both, providing the abrasive surface. Less commonly, abrasions are found involving digital pads as the consequence of prolonged exercise or contact with rough surfaces.

Complications

The mechanism of abrasion usually results in the wound becoming heavily contaminated with microorganisms and debris from the abrading surface. Moreover, the force of the abrasion ensures that these contaminants are deeply embedded in the tissue and will require careful removal during the initial stages of wound management. The debridement stage for abrasions will, therefore, often be prolonged and early wound closure is rarely a safe option. In its strictest sense, abrasion refers to a wound in which the underlying dermis remains intact and, therefore, with suitable management of the wound the dermis should be capable of providing subsequent regrowth of the epidermal layers and reconstruction will not be a consideration. For many so-called abrasion wounds, however, there is extensive tissue loss and involvement of the deeper dermal layers and the subsequent replacement or reconstruction of skin becomes an important longer term consideration.

DEGLOVING AND AVULSION WOUNDS

Aetiology

Although degloving and avulsion injuries have differing aetiologies it is convenient to discuss them together since they are often similar in appearance and have the same complications. A degloving injury describes the tearing away of skin from an extremity, usually a limb, in a manner similar to the removal of a glove from a hand. The process of degloving may be either mechanical or physiological.

Mechanical degloving, sometimes described as a stretch laceration, occurs as the overlying skin is torn from its subdermal attachments. This is most frequently seen in road traffic injuries as a car wheel runs over a limb or as the result of severe abrasive injuries (Figure 2.3).

Physiological degloving is the consequence of damage to the vascular supply as the skin and subcutaneous tissues are sheared from the deeper fascia, leading to subsequent sloughing of the overlying skin over a period of days (Figure 2.4). The aetiology of either mechanism may, however, be similar.

Avulsion injuries refer to the forcible separation of tissue from its attachments. Avulsions are commonly seen as the sequel to dog fights in which large areas of skin are simply torn from their attachments. Some of the most severe avulsions occur in dog fights and fights with badgers or foxes in which typically the dog's mandible can be extensively exposed or even removed (Figure 2.5).

Complications

Both degloving and avulsion injuries may initially be free of bacterial contamination although they may be complicated by associated orthopaedic injury. The sloughing process in physiological degloving may take several days and secondary infection of the necrotic tissue may become a problem. The major management concern is the reconstruction of what is often a large cutaneous deficit over an extremity where spare adjacent skin is at a premium. The degloved skin may remain attached by a pedicle, in which case an imme-

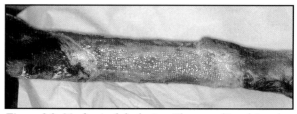

Figure 2.3: *Mechanical degloving. The wound involving the forelimb resulted from road traffic trauma. The limb was trapped under the car's wheel and the skin was stripped away between the tyre and road surface. The wound is full-circumference and was heavily contaminated with material from the road surface on initial presentation.*

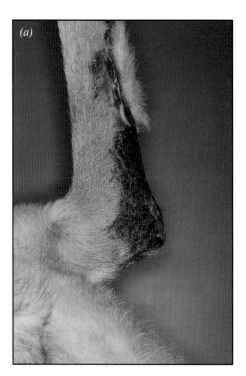

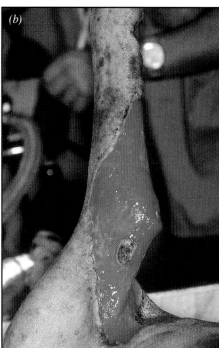

Figure 2.4: Physiological degloving. This injury was due to ischaemic damage following road traffic trauma. (a) The dog's forelimb 48 hours after the injury. Cutaneous necrosis is beginning as the result of vascular damage sustained at the time of the original injury. (b) The extent of the final area of sloughing after 7 days.

Copyright © R.A.S. White

diate reconstruction can be considered, or totally detached, in which case it can be used as a free graft. Avulsions involving the mandible represent a considerable reconstructive challenge due the difficulty of attaching skin to bone devoid of a periosteum.

SHEARING INJURIES

Aetiology

Shearing injuries have a similar aetiology to degloving wounds and are usually the result of road traffic trauma. They involve the limbs and tend to be encountered in immature dogs. The medial aspect of the carpus, phalanges and particularly the tarsometatarsal joints are particularly prone to this type of injury (Figure 2.6).

Complications

In addition to damage to the skin and associated structures, shearing wounds involve bones and, more seriously, joints. Like degloving wounds, shearing injuries are heavily contaminated with bacteria and debris from the abrading surface. These wounds are extremely prone to infection and can be expected to require long-term open wound care to prevent this. In the case of joint involvement there may be deep penetration of the joint surfaces by the contamination. The bacterial load within the joint is considered to be the major determinant for primary wound closure and most wounds should be left to heal secondarily rather than reconstructed or grafted at an early stage. Joint injuries are further complicated by the damage to their associated supporting soft tissue structures such as ligaments or tendons which gives rise to instability and occasionally valgus deformity of the carpus or tarsus.

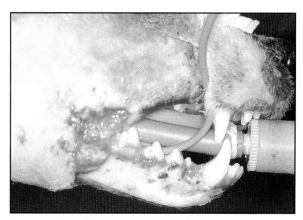

Figure 2.5: Avulsion wound. Almost the entire soft tissue covering has been removed from the ventral aspect of a terrier's mandible – the result of a confrontation with a badger.

Copyright © R.A.S. White

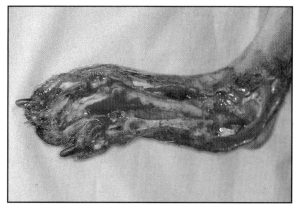

Figure 2.6: A shearing wound. There is loss of supporting soft tissue structures, exposure of the joint and deep contamination within the joint surfaces on the medial aspect of a hock.

Copyright © R.A.S. White

CAST AND BANDAGED WOUNDS

Aetiology

Wounds resulting from veterinary attention are an important and unavoidable consideration in small animal practice. Amongst the more common causes are injuries caused through poor casting or bandaging technique. Such iatrogenic wounds result from ischaemic injury following the overly tight application of the support in combination with a failure to carefully inspect the wound regularly. Thin-skinned dogs such as Greyhounds, Whippets and Lurchers are especially prone to this type of injury.

Complications

Affected areas usually involve some point of pressure (e.g. over digits, olecranon). Less serious casting wounds include sloughing of dermal layers, whilst the more serious may lead to loss of digits and even limbs (Figure 2.7). Gangrenous changes may be a further complication.

PUNCTURE WOUNDS

Aetiology

A puncture wound is the result of a sharp object moving rapidly in a plane perpendicular to the skin. A perforating wound normally refers to a puncture injury with both an entry and an exit wound, whilst a penetrating wound has only an entry wound. The most commonly encountered type of puncture wound in small animal practice is the bite injury in which the puncturing object is a tooth, particularly the canine. As the tissues are gripped, the comparatively mobile superficial layers are penetrated by the teeth whilst the fixed deeper tissues are subjected to more serious injuries due to the accompanying crushing and shearing effects. Bites may become further complicated through traction of the crushed tissues, and lacerations, contusions and separation of large areas of skin may develop.

Penetration injuries involving the oropharynx are encountered in dogs exercised by retrieving sticks. In this situation, the dog's own momentum takes it on to the stick which becomes fixed upright in the ground. These wounds may involve the tongue, the floor of the mouth, the walls of the pharynx or, in the most severe cases, the oesophagus. Less common puncture aetiologies include snake and insect bites, and firearm wounds.

Complications

Puncture wounds are characterized by a relatively small skin wound with a minimal deficit which is often of little significance in terms of wound management (Figure 2.8). However the accompanying, and often unseen, injury to the deeper tissues and the consequences of their bacterial contamination by the penetrating object are of far greater importance (Figure 2.9). The penetrating teeth may inoculate superficial tissue, including hair and bacteria from the oral cavity and skin surface, deep into the traumatized tissues. This combination of a closed wound without any natural route for drainage, contused muscle and haematoma or seroma accumulation in a dead space deprived of its normal vascular supply creates the most ideal medium possible for bacterial growth promoting rapid infection. The prevalent skin bacteria responsible for wound infections in small animals are *Staphylococcus* spp., *Streptococcus* spp. and *Pasteurella* spp., the latter predominating in the cat. However, the absence of any drainage or communication with the surface wound through the narrow wound tract, which may close prematurely, further complicates the wound by creating a hypoxic environment favouring the growth of anaerobic organisms such as *Clostridium* spp. The growth of these organisms is further assisted by their ability to inhibit neutrophil migration and to function in a region of already impoverished vascular supply (Figure 2.9). In 'little dog:big dog' confrontations the bite wounds may be severe enough to enter body

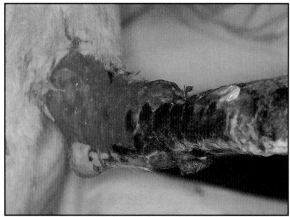

Figure 2.7: Bandage wound. Extensive full thickness skin loss following inadequate management of bandaging for a skin wound.

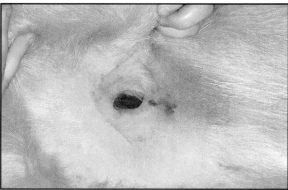

Figure 2.8: Puncture wound. A stake wound in the axilla of a dog. The modest skin injury conceals a residual length of wooden stake which has lacerated the axillary artery and brachial plexus. The traumatized environment provides an ideal medium for anaerobic bacterial growth.

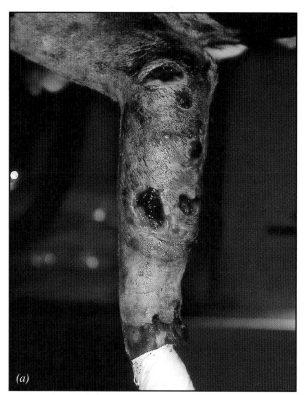

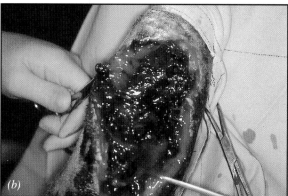

Figure 2.9: Puncture wound. A bite wound to the forearm of a dog. (a) Less than 48 hours after injury there is already gross swelling of the lower limb. (b) Surgical exploration of the wound shows widespread myonecrosis. This was due to a clostridial infection.

cavities. Here, the thoracic wounds may be complicated by rib trauma and pneumothorax, whilst abdominal wounds may be accompanied by ruptures of the abdominal wall and penetration of the viscera. Neck injuries may involve perforation of the upper airway with subcutaneous air leakage into the cervical tissues.

Stick injuries involving the floor of the mouth or pharyngeal wall cause dysphagia (Figure 2.10). Injuries involving the oesophagus are usually of a more acute and serious nature due to bacterial contamination extending to the mediastinum through the perforation (Figure 2.11). Often fragments of wood are left embedded in the wound and eventually form a septic focus which discharges via sinus tracts opening into the cervical region or into the pharynx itself.

SNAKE AND INSECT BITES/STINGS

Aetiology
Snake and insect bites are specialized forms of puncture wound which have their own specific complications as a consequence of the substances inoculated. The adder is the only venomous snake found naturally in the UK and occasionally snake bites involving an extremity are encountered in dogs exercised on areas of heath and moorland, although not all cases involve venom.

In northern Europe there are few insect species capable of causing significant wound complications, although secondary infection following incomplete removal of tick mouthparts is a well recognized problem. Wasp and bee stings may cause acute localized swelling particularly in the oral cavity.

The brown recluse spider, found in south-eastern parts of the USA, inoculates a necrotizing substance into the subcutaneous tissues, leading to serious wound complications.

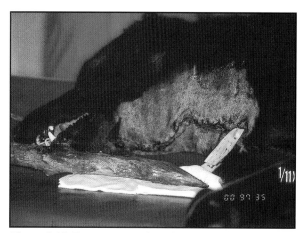

Figure 2.10: Puncture wound. A pharyngeal stick injury in the dog resulting from the dog running on to a stick thrown for retrieval by the owner. The depth of penetration is demonstrated by the stick and the exit level of the drain.

Courtesy of J M Williams.

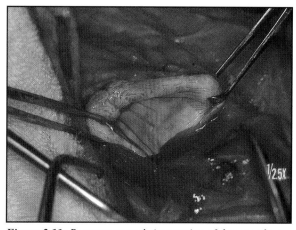

Figure 2.11: Puncture wound. Amputation of the oesophagus from its rostral attachment following a pharyngeal stick injury.

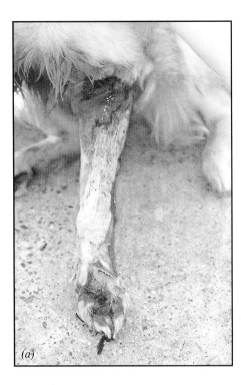

(a)

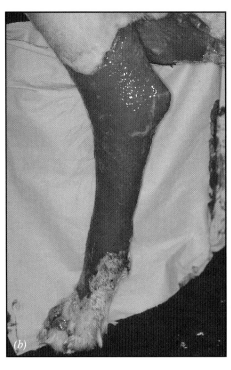

(b)

Figure 2.12: Snake bite. (a) An envenomized adder wound, resulting in widespread sloughing of the skin overlying the forelimb in a Retriever. (b) Complete loss of the skin to the forelimb 7 days after the original bite.

Copyright © R.A.S. White

Complications

Snake venom may cause a variety of both local and systemic problems. The local changes caused by adder bites include myonecrosis and damage to the blood vessel walls, leading to ischaemia and tissue sloughing (Figure 2.12). The venom inoculated by the brown recluse spider is capable of causing extensive and alarmingly rapid tissue necrosis, confined initially to the skin and subcutaneous structures, but in some cases this can severe enough to cause the loss of a digit or even a limb.

BURNS

Aetiology

Burns are injuries caused by an extreme of heat or cold or by another physical agent having a similar effect, e.g. electricity, caustic agents or radiation.

Thermal burns

Thermal burns are the consequence of extremes of heat (hyperthermic) or cold (hypothermic). As a general comment, the small animal species seem remarkably less prone than their human counterparts to this type of wounding. Hyperthermic burns may be the result of: scalds; contact with hot surfaces (car exhaust during road traffic injuries); or malicious immersion in, followed by ignition of, flammable fluids. Classically, scalds are encountered involving either the dorsum or ventrum of the animal. Dorsal scalds are the result of domestic accidents involving boiling water or fat being tipped over the animal; ventral scalds are seen in animals which are either dropped, or not uncommonly jump, into boiling water. Recumbent patients left for

prolonged periods on faulty or badly monitored heating beds during surgery or in intensive care units may sustain iatrogenic burns (Figure 2.13). Hypothermic burns occur through frostbite and usually involve the extremities (tail tips, pinnae and nose). Although uncommon in the UK, they are encountered more frequently in the northern parts of the European and American continents.

Chemical burns

Chemical burns result from contact with caustic materials such as battery acid, alkalis and phenol. The wounds may involve the footpads or, in cases of ingestion, there may be oropharyngeal and oesophageal burning.

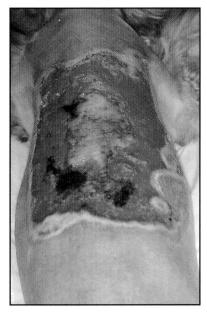

Figure 2.13: Burn. An iatrogenic hyperthermic injury caused by a hot water bottle being placed in direct contact with the patient's dorsum during a routine mastectomy procedure.

Copyright © R.A.S. White

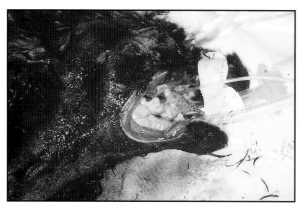

Figure 2.14: Burn. An electrical contact burn in a young puppy that chewed through a live electrical wire. Notice the extent of the lip wound and exposure of the mandible. There was additional damage to the tongue and to the hard palate.

Copyright © R.A.S. White

Electrical burns

Electrical burns can result from the animal touching a low-tension electrical source (contact burns) or from indirect contact with a high-tension source (flash or arc burns). Contact burns result from the current passing into the body and commonly are the result of puppies chewing through unearthed electrical cables (Figure 2.14). Flash burns are superficial thermal injuries seen occasionally in animals coming close to high-voltage cables (e.g. railway lines) as the current is earthed.

Radiation burns

Radiation burns can result from exposure to doses of irradiation greater than 40–50 Gy, depending on the radiation tolerance of the irradiated tissue. Tissue overlying bone appears to be particularly prone to this type of burn. Rarely a problem in everyday practice, radiation burns can pose considerable complications in the oncological patient.

Complications

The problems associated with burns in small animals are poorly understood (see Chapter 12). Burns have been classically described according to their depth:

First degree burn:	involves only the epidermis
Second degree burn:	epidermis and variable depth of the dermis
Third degree burn:	entire skin thickness +/− underlying tissues.

This classification has been gradually abandoned, although estimation of the affected proportion of the patient's surface area remains an important descriptive method.

Much information has been incorrectly extrapolated from experience with human burn patients and it is evident there are several very important differences. In particular, it is quite clear that small animals can sustain burns to relatively large surface areas (>50%) without experiencing the severe systemic and metabolic complications common in human burn patients. Nevertheless, these complications may be recognized in the small animal patient and include dehydration, hyper/hyponatraemia, hyper/hypokalaemia, acidosis, azotaemia and anaemia, and pulmonary oedema resulting from smoke inhalation.

Although secondary infection of the wound is common, septicaemia is an unusual complication. Burnt tissue often shows a distinct line of demarcation at its junction with the healthy surrounding tissue within a few hours. Early resection of the devitalized area with immediate reconstruction is now considered preferable to the practice of retaining the eschar *in situ*. In addition to shortening the period of wound management it also helps to limit the potential for the other serious long-term complication associated with burn wounds, namely, scarring (Figure 2.15). First degree burns normally heal without major cosmetic change but second degree burns will result in scarring whilst in third degree injuries all layers of the skin will have been destroyed requiring reconstruction. All scars and grafts tend to contract and there is the potential for loss of limb function through contracture of the overlying tissues.

Electrical contact burns are most often seen in young puppies that chew through unearthed cables. The consequences can be extremely serious; initially this is because the burn may involve or completely destroy lips, tongue, palate or mandible and create severe feeding problems. Secondly, the burnt tissues are immature and easily damaged and their reconstruction in the longer term is complex. Flash burns usually involve a limb or other extremity and, although they may pose serious reconstruction problems, they are less likely to be accompanied by such severe damage to underlying structures.

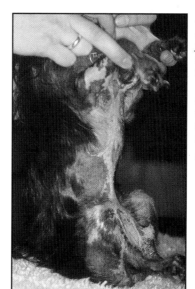

Figure 2.15: Burn. Extensive scarring following an immersion scald injury. Note the 'webbing' of the axillae, groin and ventrum, causing severe restriction of orthopaedic function.

Copyright © R.A.S. White

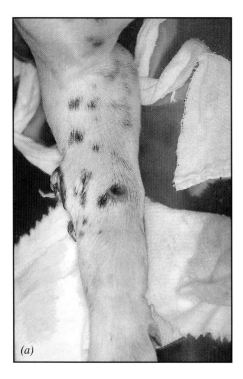

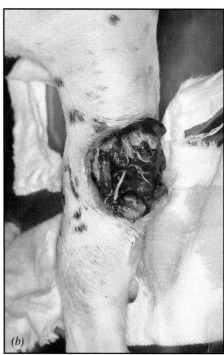

Figure 2.16: Firearm wound. A high-velocity ballistic wound involving the forelimb of a dog that was shot by a 0.223 calibre military weapon. (a) The entry wound is small, round and regular with little indication of the underlying trauma. (b) The size of the exit wound emphasizes the conical shape of the wound caused by the shockwave of the impacting ballistic. The distal two-thirds of the radius and ulna had been removed by the shockwave through the exit wound.

Copyright © R.A.S. White

FIREARM INJURIES

Aetiology

The mechanics of firearm wounds is complex and far beyond this brief discussion (see Chapter 12). It is convenient to categorize firearm injuries according to the type of weapon involved, since the pattern of trauma is determined in the first instance by the velocity of the missile. As the velocity of the missile increases, so the kinetic energy which it is capable of imparting to the impacted tissue increases exponentially:

$$\text{Kinetic Energy} = \frac{\text{Mass x Velocity}^2}{2\,g}$$

where g = acceleration due to gravity.

Missiles from shotguns, airguns and handguns have a muzzle velocity of <300 m/s and are regarded as being of *low velocity*. Hunting rifle projectiles have muzzle velocities of 300–800 m/s and are classified as *medium velocity*, whilst military rifle missiles travel at >1000 m/s and are considered as *high velocity*.

Complications

The entry and exit wounds of low-velocity missiles are generally of small diameter and the tissue tract has a regular diameter. In the case of shotgun wounds the proximity of the weapon and resulting density of missile spread also determine the type of entry wound and may result in extensive removal of skin and associated tissues. The deeper tissues are traumatized mainly by laceration and compression, leaving a regular diameter (i.e. cylindrical) tract with comparatively minor damage.

Medium- and high-velocity missiles traumatize tissue by imparting their kinetic energy to the surrounding tissues, causing a compression wave which moves ahead of the ballistic. This energy is converted either into stretching forces within the tissue or to disruption creating cavitation of the tissues. The greater the velocity, the greater the tendency to cavitation. Entry wounds may be modest but exit wounds are large (Figure 2.16). The severity of the wound pattern is further influenced by the type of ballistic. Expanding bullets extend the size of the cavity, as does any tendency for the bullet to 'tumble' through the tissues causing an expanding (i.e. conical) tract (see Chapter 12).

FURTHER READING

Beardsley SL and Schrader SC (1995) Treatment of dogs with wounds of the limbs caused by shearing forces: 98 cases (1975-1993). *Journal of the American Veterinary Medical Association* **207**, 1071-1075

Kolata RJ and Burrows CF (1981) The clinical features of injury by chewing electrical cords in dogs and cats. *Journal of the American Animal Hospital Association* **17**, 219-222

Pavletic MM (1986) Gunshot wounds in veterinary medicine: projectile ballistics. Part 1. *Compendium on Continuing Education for the Practicing Veterinarian* **8**, 47-60

Pavletic MM (1986) Gunshot wounds in veterinary medicine: projectile ballistics. Part 2. *Compendium on Continuing Education for the Practicing Veterinarian* **8**, 125-134

Pope ER (1993) Burns: thermal, electrical, chemical and cold injuries. In: *Textbook of Small Animal Surgery, 2nd edn*, ed. DH Slatter, pp.355-369. WB Saunders, Philadelphia

Renegar WR and Stoll SG (1980) Gunshot wounds involving the canine carpus: surgical management. *Journal of the American Animal Hospital Association* **16**, 233-239

CHAPTER THREE

Wound Healing and Influencing Factors

Clare R. Gregory

THE PRINCIPLES OF WOUND HEALING

The phrase 'wound healing' is often used exclusively to describe the process that occurs in the skin as the body restores the integrity of lost tissue by the formation of a collagenous scar. However, similar processes to those that occur in the skin also occur during repair in a variety of other tissues and organs. This repair may represent maintenance of wear and tear injuries that occur in joints, replacement of highly proliferative cells with short life spans, such as epithelial cells lining the intestinal tract, or the repair of traumatic injuries.

Injury of any type triggers an organized and complex cascade of cellular and biochemical events that result in a healed wound. These processes can lead to pathological conditions if healing is excessive or deficient. Wound healing failures can pose a significant clinical problem with a large impact on morbidity, mortality and medical costs. A grasp of the fundamental physiology of wound healing results in a better understanding of the pathophysiological processes that impair wound healing.

The wound healing process is often divided into three overlapping phases:

1. Haemostasis and inflammation
2. Proliferation
3. Maturation and remodelling.

Haemostasis and inflammation

Traumatic injuries, such as those caused by road traffic accidents or gunshots, account for many wounds in domestic animals. Other wounding factors include physical agents such as heat and cold, chemicals, ionizing radiation, microbial infection, neoplasia and surgical intervention. Haemorrhage occurs to varying degrees in all wounds and must be controlled. The rupture of vessels exposes the subendothelial collagen to platelets and results in aggregation of platelets and the activation of the intrinsic part of the coagulation cascade. The contact between collagen and platelets, as well as the presence of thrombin, fibronectin and their fragments, results in the release of cytokines and growth factors from platelets and the surrounding

tissues. Although the locally formed fibrin clot (Figure 3.1) is important for temporarily sealing the wound and for providing a lattice framework for subsequent migration of neutrophils, monocytes, fibroblasts and endothelial cells, it is also an impediment to wound healing. It increases the amount of devitalized cellular debris that must be removed by inflammatory and cellular processes, it enlarges wound dead space and it provides an excellent medium for microbial growth.

The migration of cells into the injured tissue appears to occur in sequence. Increased vascular permeability and release of prostaglandins, together with the release of chemotactic substances such as complement factors, interleukin-1, tumour necrosis factor-α (TNF-α), transforming growth factor-β (TGF-β), platelet factor 4 and bacterial products, stimulate neutrophil migration within hours of wounding. Neutrophils are followed by monocytes, lymphocytes and fibroblasts. All cells participating in wound healing must be activated. Activation entails the phenotypic altering of cellular, biochemical and functional properties induced by local physical and biochemical mediators. Activation may induce new cell surface antigen expression, increased cytotoxicity, or increased production and release of cytokines and growth factors. Neutrophils, macrophages and lymphocytes predominate during inflammation, but the contribution of each cell population to the successful outcome of wound healing is variable. Macrophages and lymphocytes exert critical roles, but neutrophils are not essential, provided that no bacterial contamination is present, since their role in phagocytosis and antimicrobial defence may be taken over by macrophages.

In contrast, healing is severely impaired when macrophage function is suppressed. The activation of macrophages has fundamental implications in several areas of wound healing including debridement, matrix synthesis and angiogenesis. Wound macrophages are derived from blood monocytes that migrate into injured tissue. The initial release of chemotactic and growth factors from platelets is the first stimulus, and a strong one, of macrophage activation. The phagocytosis of cellular debris such as fibronectin or collagen also contributes to their activation. This activation also leads to the release of additional cytokines and

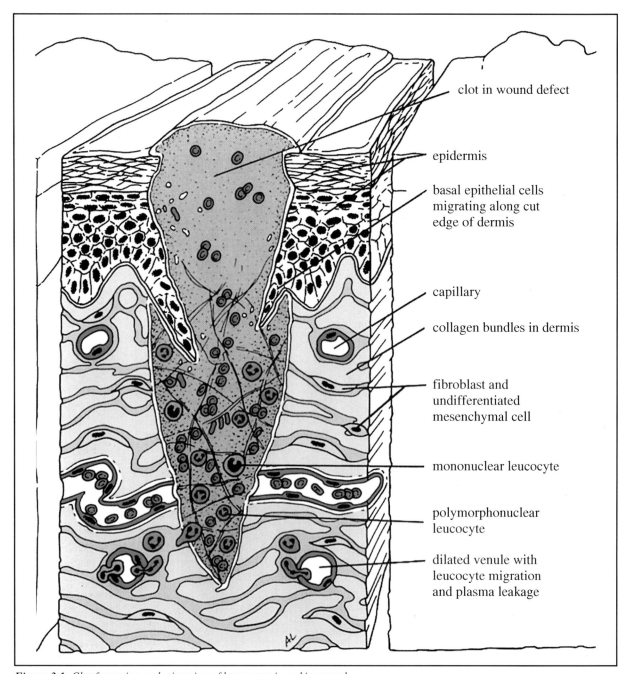

clot in wound defect

epidermis

basal epithelial cells migrating along cut edge of dermis

capillary

collagen bundles in dermis

fibroblast and undifferentiated mesenchymal cell

mononuclear leucocyte

polymorphonuclear leucocyte

dilated venule with leucocyte migration and plasma leakage

Figure 3.1: Clot formation and migration of leucocytes in a skin wound.

Reproduced from Pascoe (1992) with permission.

nitric oxide (NO), which mediate angiogenesis and fibroplasia. Activated macrophages can activate other cells such as lymphocytes via cytokines which, in turn, release lymphokines (interferons, interleukins) that act back on macrophages to release additional cytokines such as TNF-α and interleukin-1 (IL-1). This interaction ensures a prolonged presence of cytokines in the wound bed and illustrates the network of interactions between cells during healing. The rate of production and the half-life of these chemotactic factors and cytokines directly regulate macrophage function and modulate the healing process (Figure 3.2).

The primary function of the fibroblast is to synthesize and deposit proteoglycans and collagen,

the principal components of the extracellular connective tissue matrix. Wound fibroblasts are thought to be derived from pluripotential perivascular mesenchymal cells and from local tissue fibroblasts. The stimulus for the phenotypic alteration or activation of wound fibroblasts originates mainly from macrophage-derived cytokines such as TGF-β, epidermal growth factor (EGF) and platelet derived growth factor (PDGF). The matrix surrounding the cells, such as the presence of fibronectin, tissue oxygen content and acidity, also influences their activation.

While the inflammatory responses to wounding result in a marked cellular response within hours to days,

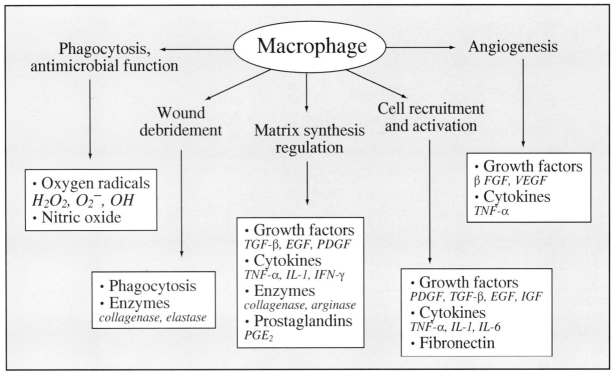

Figure 3.2: *The central role of the macrophage in wound healing.*

Reproduced from Witte and Barbol (1992) with the permission of WB Saunders.

diminished inflammatory responses and suppressing fibroblastic activity profoundly limit subsequent healing. For example, reduced inflammation induced by corticosteroid administration decreases cell migration, proliferation and subsequent angiogenesis.

Proliferation

Approximately 24–36 hours after wounding, fibroblasts and endothelial cells adjacent to the wound margins begin to divide and multiply. The growth factors and cytokines responsible for the proliferation of these two cell types are derived mainly from platelets and activated macrophages. Some are stored in the matrix of the fibrin clot which is invaded by the cells. Fibroblasts and endothelial cells can also be activated to release additional growth factors which act in an autocrine manner. Endothelial cells proliferate from intact venules close to the wound and form new capillaries by the process of angiogenesis. Endothelial buds develop on these capillaries and grow towards the leading edge in an arcuate pattern (Figure 3.3). Each endothelial bud unites with another endothelial bud in an open wound, with a cut vessel in a skin graft, or with another vessel on the opposite side of a surgically apposed incision. After fusion, the endothelial bud is canalized and spasmodic blood flow begins. Mitotic activity in adjacent mesenchymal cells increases as a regular blood flow is established. As the vascular network advances, the connective tissue cells left behind become more clearly recognizable as fibroblasts.

Neutrophils and lymphocytes undergo apoptosis and are ingested by macrophages. The connective tissue spaces that were initially filled with proteoglycans, protocollagen and tropocollagen begin to display clearly differentiated, thin collagen fibrils lying parallel to the longitudinal axis of the fibroblasts. Growing between the immature fibroblasts, the developing capillaries are surrounded by tropocollagen, which condenses to form a supporting framework of collagen fibrils. As healing continues, many of the earlier capillaries transform into larger vessels or stop functioning and disappear. Lymphatic channels develop in a manner that is similar to, but much slower than, blood vessels, so that lymphatic drainage of the wound is poor during early wound healing.

The tissue that fills the wound space, called granulation tissue, is a mixture of branching capillary loops surrounded by mesenchymal cells and extracellular matrix. This tissue is highly resistant to infection because of the zone of granulocytes and macrophages on its outer surface. Granulation tissue does not usually grow beyond the surface of any organ, especially if the epithelial regeneration that has been occurring simultaneously is complete.

Maturation and remodelling

Restoration of tissue continuity after injury and the strength of the ensuing repair tissue depend almost entirely on the period of fibroplasia. Additional tensile strength develops during the maturation and

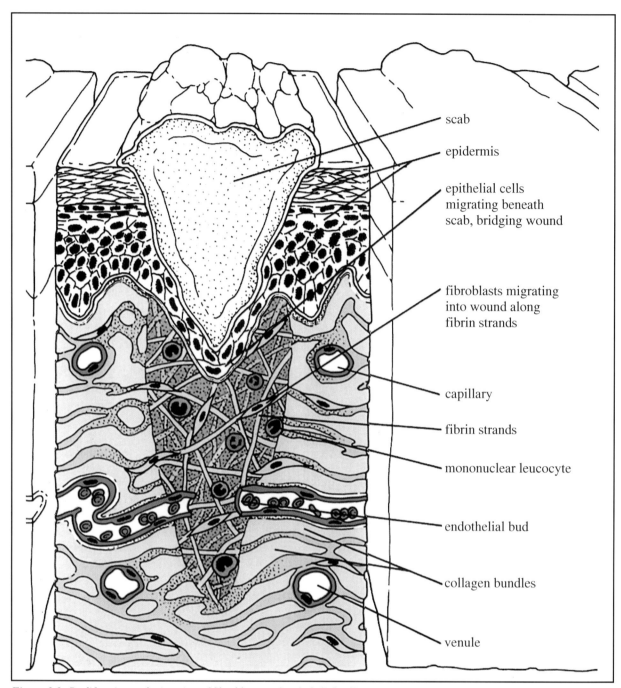

scab

epidermis

epithelial cells
migrating beneath
scab, bridging wound

fibroblasts migrating
into wound along
fibrin strands

capillary

fibrin strands

mononuclear leucocyte

endothelial bud

collagen bundles

venule

Figure 3.3: *Proliferation and migration of fibroblasts and endothelial cells.*

Reproduced from Pascoe (1992) with permission.

remodelling phase as the new collagen undergoes structural modification. From a clinical viewpoint, this is the most important phase of wound healing because the rate, quality and total amount of matrix deposition determine the strength of the scar. This period begins about 15 days after wounding and can continue for many months depending on the tissue involved, being prolonged in tendon healing. After granulation tissue fills the defect, there is a gradual diminution in the number of synthesizing fibroblasts, a regression of the capillary network, and a decline in the rate of collagen synthesis until it balances the rate of collagen breakdown.

There is a slow, steady increase in wound tensile strength due to the gradual intermolecular and intramolecular cross-linking of the tropocollagen molecules and the remodelling, dissolution and reformation of collagen fibres, which produce a stronger, more efficient weave. Generally, the collagen fibres remaining in a scar are oriented along lines of tension, but the scar that is formed is rarely as strong as the tissue it has replaced. After 1 week, the wound has only 3%, and after 3 weeks, 20% of its final strength. After 3 months it has approximately 80% of the strength of unwounded skin, but there is no further increase thereafter.

Wound contraction

Wound contraction is the reduction of part or all of a defect by movement of the normal surrounding tissue towards the centre of the defect. Wound contraction is the approximation of the wound edges and wound contracture is the shortening of the scar itself. Several theories have been proposed for the mechanisms of wound contraction. One suggests that a special cell, the myofibroblast, is responsible for contraction, leading the skin edge across the wound. Another theory suggests that the locomotion of all fibroblasts leads to a reorganization of the matrix and to contraction. Wound contraction starts almost immediately following wounding and continues for 2–3 weeks.

Healing skin wounds are readily distorted when the skin on one side of a defect is less mobile than the skin on the opposite side. Distortions that produce an undesirable cosmetic effect are common with facial wounds, particularly those involving the eyelids, lips and ears. Contraction of wounds involving the skin and soft tissue structures around joints may also result in structural deformities of limbs with subsequent impairment or loss of function. In tubular organs like the digestive tract, contraction may result in shortening or stricture of the organ. Contraction may stop before the defect is obliterated if the surrounding skin tension exceeds the contractile force of the granulation tissue, or if myofibroblast development or function is impaired. Contraction may be impaired by the administration of corticosteroids, by antimicrotubular drugs and by the local application of smooth muscle relaxants. Mechanical splinting of open wounds only inhibits contraction until the splints are removed. Split-thickness skin grafts may occasionally slow con-traction, but full-thickness skin grafts or skin flaps markedly inhibit contraction.

Epithelialization

Epithelial surfaces provide an important barrier to external infection and internal fluid loss. In linear and superficial epithelial wounds, epithelial regeneration usually covers the wound before new connective tissue forms. In deeper open wounds in which there is extensive loss of basement membrane and underlying connective tissue, epithelial repair occurs in concert with the development of new connective tissue. The surface area of newly formed epithelium is then gradually reduced as the underlying granulation tissue contracts. Epidermal repair involves the mobilization, migration, proliferation and differentiation of epithelial cells (Figure 3.4). Migrating epithelial cells lose many of their desmosomal attachments to the basement membrane and to other epithelial cells. Basal cells at the wound edge develop microvilli and extend broad, thin pseudopodia over the exposed surface of the collagen bundles. Epithelial cells in the layers behind the basal cells migrate over them until contact with the wound surface is made. This process continues with cells from the proliferating edge sliding forward over the attached cells until the surface is covered.

After the basement membrane is established, the epithelial cells proliferate to restore the normal columnar architecture of stratified squamous epithelium (Figure 3.5). Cellular differentiation occurs, characterized by keratinization of the outer cell layers. The intense cellular activity that produces epithelial cells and makes them ready for migration occurs within 2–5 mm of the wound margin. About 10 days after wounding, epithelial projections grow down into the underlying connective tissue. These epithelial spurs regress by the 36th day following wounding leaving the basal border of the regenerated epidermis relatively smooth. Once the new epidermis has been established, the rate of cell division rapidly declines, and the epidermal thickness is reduced. The epidermis over the wound often remains several cells thicker than the surrounding epidermis for at least a year.

The route and rate of epithelial migration depend on the environment of the wound. Because the epithelial cells only migrate over viable tissue, they must move beneath a scab or eschar. Epithelial cell migration and mitosis appear to be maximized when the wound environment is moist, devoid of both infection and eschar, protected with an oxygen-permeable membrane, and exposed to hyperbaric oxygen. In clinical practice, optimum epithelial repair occurs in a moist, well oxygenated environment without eschar or infection. The use of wet-to-dry dressings, although effective in debriding necrotic tissue in wounds, is often detrimental to epithelial repair. The moist environment encourages epithelial repair, but the newly formed epithelium is also debrided as the dried dressing is removed.

Wherever suture material penetrates the epidermis or epidermal appendages, epithelial migration occurs along the suture tract. Once the tract is lined with epithelium, proliferation and keratinization may produce a foreign body reaction, sterile abscess and a scar. In most situations, this type of scarring is relatively unimportant in domestic animals because of their coat of hair.

In full-thickness open skin wounds, epithelial migration occurs only from the wound margins. If islands of dermis containing transected adnexal structures (hair follicles and sebaceous glands) or islands of full-thickness skin remain, there is epithelial migration from these structures as well as from the wound margins.

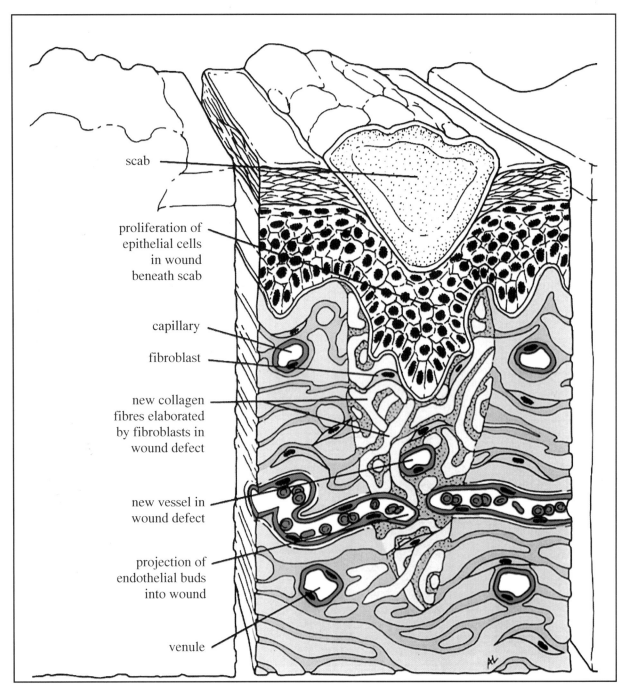

Figure 3.4: *Mobilization, migration, proliferation and differentiation of epithelial cells.*

Reproduced from Pascoe (1992) with permission.

FACTORS THAT INFLUENCE WOUND HEALING

Traditional influences

Local factors that influence wound healing include:

- The surgical technique and experience of the surgeon
- The quality of the vascular supply to the area
- The presence of a deleterious infection
- Mechanical stress on the wound
- Abrasive or inflammatory suture material
- Radiation injury.

Systemic factors that influence wound healing include:

- Hypoproteinaemia and hypovolaemia
- Oedema
- Malnutrition and vitamin deficiency
- The administration of corticosteroids
- Diabetes mellitus
- The administration of cytotoxic drugs
- Jaundice
- Uraemia
- Advanced age.

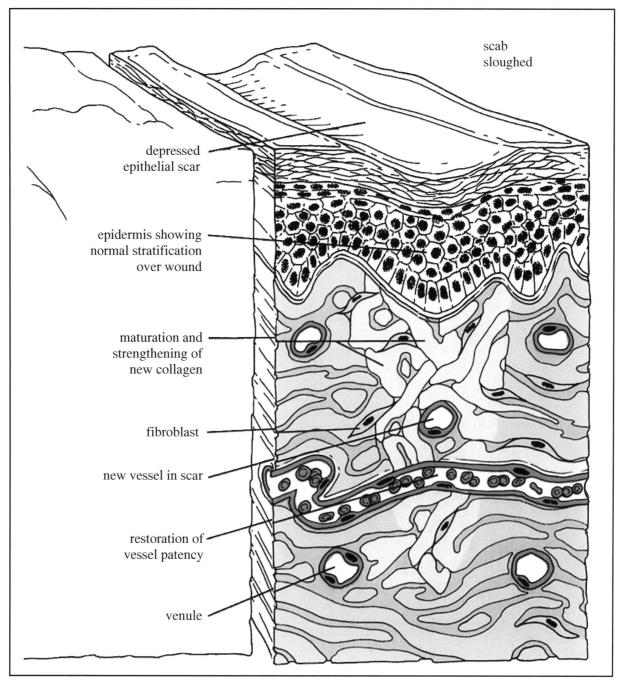

scab
sloughed

depressed
epithelial scar

epidermis showing
normal stratification
over wound

maturation and
strengthening of
new collagen

fibroblast

new vessel in scar

restoration of
vessel patency

venule

Figure 3.5: *Final remodelling stages with normal epidermal stratification and maturation of new collagen.*

Reproduced from Pascoe (1992) with permission.

The essentials of good surgical technique that can avoid delays in wound healing include the following:

- Minimizing wound trauma by gentle tissue handling and decreasing the duration of the procedure
- Thorough debridement and removal of foreign bodies to minimize contamination and to reduce the possibility of infection
- Meticulous haemostasis to prevent haematoma and seroma formation, while maintaining the vascular supply of the tissue

- Avoiding tissue necrosis from excessive use of ligatures or cautery
- Minimizing dead space by close approximation of tissue layers
- Minimizing mechanical stress (tension) on wound edges
- Selection of appropriate suture materials and suturing techniques.

Infection slows gain of wound strength in animal studies. Corticosteroids are known to affect healing adversely, particularly due to a lack in the development of tensile strength. A variety of cytotoxic drugs also delay gain in wound tensile strength. It is customary to delay administration of an antineoplastic agent in a postoperative cancer patient until the acute healing phase is over, usually 2–3 weeks. Skin wounds in animals that receive a radiation dose within 2 days after wounding have 50% of the strength of control incisions at 7 and 14 days. The effect of radiation on healing when administered 1 week or more after wounding is probably negligible. Tissue irradiated prior to surgery often heals poorly because of its inadequate blood supply. Malnutrition, hypoproteinaemia and anaemia have been shown to delay wound healing in many animal models.

Peptide growth factors

The purpose of this section is to give a brief introduction to a very rapidly expanding area of biology: the acceleration of tissue healing in normal and physiologically compromised wounds. This section will introduce the five major families of peptide growth factors currently under study. The names of most will come and go as their expectation does not meet clinical needs, but a few will be successful and will probably be a common item on the shelf of the veterinary pharmacy in a few years.

Peptide growth factors play a key role in initiating and sustaining wound healing. Platelets degranulate and release PDGF, TGF-β, EGF and insulin-like growth factor-1 (IGF-1). These substances stimulate the chemotaxis of inflammatory cells, fibroblasts, epithelial cells, and vascular endothelial cells. As mentioned above, growth factors released from inflammatory cells, fibroblasts, macrophages, epithelial cells and others sustain the wound healing process: in growth of blood vessels, formation of collagen and formation of secondary glands and structures.

Peptide growth factors stimulate the continuous mitosis of quiescent cells in complete media that lack serum. They are synthesized and secreted by many types of cells. Growth factors can act on the producer cell (autocrine), adjacent cells (paracrine, juxtacrine) or on distant cells (endocrine). Growth factors all act by binding to and activating specific, high affinity receptor proteins on the cell membranes of target cells. However, growth factors are rapidly degraded by proteases.

Five families of growth factors are currently recognized for their potential role in wound healing: epithelial growth factor (EGF), transforming growth factor beta (TGF-β), insulin-like growth factor (IGF), platelet-derived growth factor (PDGF) and fibroblast growth factor (FGF).

Epithelial growth factor (EGF)

EGF is synthesized by renal cells, lacrimal glands, salivary glands and megakaryocytes. It is found in tears, saliva and urine. EGF promotes healing by stimulating migration and division of epithelial cells.

It increases the synthesis of proteins such as fibronectin that aid in cell attachment and migration. EGF has been shown to accelerate epidermal regeneration in pig skin, and corneal lesions in rabbits and primates. Wounds treated with EGF show increasing numbers of fibroblasts and a larger scar area. In human clinical trials, EGF increased epidermal regeneration of dermatome wounds, increased the healing in chronic wounds and promoted epithelialization of corneal wounds.

Transforming growth factor beta (TGF-β)

TGF-β is synthesized by platelets, macrophages, lymphocytes, fibroblasts, bone cells and keratinocytes. Nearly all cells have TGF-β receptors. TGF-β inhibits the growth of several types of cells including smooth muscle cells and leucocytes, but it is mitogenic for fibroblasts. It is stored in a latent form and requires activation by plasmin or low pH. In wounds, TGF-β stimulates the chemotaxis of inflammatory cells and stimulates the synthesis of extracellular matrix; it may be the most important regulatory peptide in wound healing.

We studied the effectiveness of TGF-β for the healing of chronic soft tissue wounds that had not healed, or were not expected to heal, using standard therapies. Biopsies of several wounds were taken, both prior to and following treatment. After cleansing, TGF-β (0.1 mg/ml in 3% methyl cellulose) was applied topically, once daily, every 3 days in volumes ranging from 0.1 to 0.5 ml. The following are examples of the animals treated and the results.

Case One
Golden Retriever, female, ovariohysterectomized, 7 years old
Diagnosis: Immune-mediated polyarthritis
Treatment: Prednisolone and amoxicillin
Problem: Full thickness ulceration of the skin over the left elbow joint
Further treatment: Prednisolone therapy was continued. Four weeks after the initiation of TGF-β therapy, the elbow lesion was healed. The wound remained healed 9 weeks after TGF-β therapy was discontinued.

Case Two
Golden Retriever, female, ovariohysterectomized, 6 years old
Diagnosis: Osteosarcoma of the radius
Treatment: Limb sparing using a cortical allograft and intralesional cisplatin
Problem: Full thickness skin ulcer over the allograft; 5 week duration. A biopsy of the wound edge revealed necrotic connective tissue and epidermal hyperplasia
Further treatment: Intravenous cisplatin was continued. Three weeks following the initiation of TGF-β therapy, the wound was healed.

Case Three

Tibetan Terrier, female, ovariohysterectomized, 9 years old

Diagnosis: Immune-mediated dermatitis and iatrogenic hyperadrenocorticism

Treatment: Prednisolone and azathioprine

Problem: Full thickness ulceration of many footpads

Further treatment: Prednisolone and azathioprine treatment continued. Eight weeks following initiation of TGF-β therapy, all pad lesions were healed except for one, a 1 x 1 mm lesion. A biopsy from the healing pad lesion revealed fibroplasia, despite immunosuppressive therapy, and bacterial infection.

Case Four

Golden eagle, adult, male

Diagnosis: Self-inflicted injury to the left wing with both tendon and bone exposed

Treatment: The wound was 75% healed at $6^1/_2$ weeks following the initiation of TGF-β therapy and treatment was discontinued. The wound went on to heal completely.

Case Five

Asian elephant, female, 36 years old

Problem: A 28-year history of a full thickness skin ulcer, approximately 8 cm in diameter, over the left hip

Treatment: The wound was 75% healed following 8 weeks of therapy and completely granulated and covered following 12 weeks of therapy.

In these cases, TGF-β appeared to accelerate the healing of soft tissue wounds; it was effective in patients with immune-mediated disease that were receiving immunosuppressive therapy. In all cases, TGF-β was effective in the presence of infection in the wound bed.

Insulin-like growth factor (IGF)

IGF is found in two forms: IGF1, which is secreted by cells of the brain, liver, heart, lung, kidney, pancreas, cartilage and muscle; and IGF2, which is more important in fetal development. IGF is reversibly bound by high-affinity IGF binding proteins in the serum; only free IGF is active. It is a potent chemotactic agent for vascular endothelial cells and results in increased neovascularization, it stimulates the mitosis of fibroblasts, osteocytes and chrondrocytes and it enhances dermal and epidermal regeneration. IGF secretion is stimulated by growth hormone. They work in concert: together they stimulate skeletal cartilage and bone growth, and increase organ size. IGF has been shown to stimulate thymic regrowth and improve T lymphocyte function. In our laboratory, IGF1 promoted thymic growth in young cats and increased T cell function in cats with feline immunodeficiency syndrome.

Platelet-derived growth factor (PDGF) and vascular endothelial growth factor (VEGF)

PDGF and VEGF are in the same family. PDGF is secreted by platelets, placental cells, fibroblasts, smooth muscle cells, vascular endothelial cells and macrophages. It is a potent chemotactic agent for macrophages and smooth muscle cells and is an early promoter of cell migration and fibrogenesis. PDGF causes increased granulation tissue formation in diabetic cats and increased healing of pressure ulcers in human patients.

Fibroblast growth factor (FGF)

FGF is bound by heparin in the extracellular matrix of most tissues; bound FGF is protected from proteolysis. It is thought that the release of heparinase, cathepsin D and collagenase by tissue injury causes the release of FGF. It is a mitogen for endothelial cells, fibroblasts, keratinocytes, chrondrocytes and smooth muscle cells. In animal models it induces cell migration, neovascularization and formation of granulation tissue. FGF is produced by fibroblasts, astrocytes, endothelium, smooth muscle cells, chrondrocytes, macrophages and osteoblasts.

All the recognized peptide growth factors appear to work in concert in wound healing. Little is understood about the initiation, control or inhibition of their actions. Growth factors are also implicated in pathological situations, where their effects have a detrimental effect (e.g. coronary vascular disease, renal fibrosis, exuberant scar formation). Many clinical trials will have to be performed before the exact indications for the use of growth factors are known. In preliminary work, it appears that growth factors, especially TGF-β, are effective in accelerating wound healing in immunosuppressed patients and others that have compromised healing.

The role of anti-growth factors in modifying tissue healing

Over the last several years, many investigators have been seeking new, more effective and less toxic immunosuppressive agents. Cyclosporin led the way by demonstrating two important facts: 1) immunosuppression can be specific to cells of the immune system; and 2) immunosuppressive agents can be profitable. The specific mechanism of action of cyclosporin also led to a rapid advancement in the understanding of T cell activation and the interrelated roles of macrophages, platelets, cytokines and growth factors in the organ and tissue rejection response. Understanding the underlying cellular and subcellular events that produce graft rejection led to the search for agents that could specifically interrupt one or more elements of the rejection process.

Chronic graft rejection is a complex process that ultimately results in failure of the transplanted organ. Unlike acute rejection, chronic rejection can progress for months to years, often undetected. In all organs, two lesions stand out: fibrosis of the interstitial areas with loss of native architecture, and occlusion of arteries and/or bronchioles by proliferating smooth muscle cells and extracellular matrix. This arterial intimal thickening results in regional hypoxia, ischaemia and tissue death. The cause of chronic rejection is unknown, but it is associated with ongoing immune injury, acute rejection episodes, prolonged warm ischaemia times and a small donor to large recipient relationship. It appears to be a low-grade, chronic ongoing inflammatory process marked by inappropriate fibrosis and vascular occlusion.

Smooth muscle cell proliferation and migration can also be seen following balloon catheter angioplasty performed for the correction of vascular narrowing caused by atherosclerosis. Many types of trauma result in arterial intimal thickening: mechanical trauma, chemical trauma, ischaemic injury and immune injury have all produced arterial intimal thickening. In each case smooth muscle cell proliferation and migration and the production of extracellular matrix is thought to be mediated by growth factors and cytokines (e.g. PDGF, FGF, IL-1, TGF-β, interferon-γ, RANTES) that are released by activated platelets, injured endothelial cells, smooth muscle cells, macrophages and from the extracellular matrix.

In addition to studying the anti-T cell effects of various potential immunosuppressive agents, our laboratories began to study the effects of each agent on growth factor-induced smooth muscle cell proliferation, and on *in vivo* models of arterial intimal thickening. Our goal was to find safe, effective immunosuppressive agents that might have the potential to reduce the incidence of chronic rejection. The following is a discussion of three agents that are currently in clinical trials for the control of allograft rejection or for the treatment of rheumatoid arthritis. Each agent may prove extremely useful for the control of wound healing or to minimize fibrosis.

Sirolimus

This is also known as RPM. It is a natural microbial substance produced by the actinomycete *Streptomyces hygroscopicus*. RPM is a hydrophobic macrocyclic lactone. It passes through cell membranes easily and binds to a cytosolic binding protein, FKBP. RPM suppresses protein synthesis in T cells, and this effect may be related to the inhibition of a kinase, 70-kDa S6 kinase, which increases the protein synthetic activity of the S6 ribosomal protein. While cyclosporin and FK506 block the T cell cycle progression at G_o - G_1, RPM prevents cells from progressing from G_1 to the S phase of the cell cycle. RPM also directly inhibits B cell immunoglobulin synthesis caused by interleukins. RPM's antagonism of cytokine and growth factor action is not limited to cells of the immune system.

Growth factor-induced proliferation of fibroblasts, endothelial cells, hepatocytes and smooth muscle cells is inhibited by RPM. Molecule for molecule, RPM has been the most effective antiproliferative agent tested in our laboratories in both *in vitro* and *in vivo* models of arterial intimal thickening.

Mycophenolic acid

Mycophenolate mofetil is a prodrug which, when hydrolysed by liver esterases, produces the active metabolite, mycophenolic acid (MPA). MPA is a non-competitive, reversible inhibitor of IMPDH, an enzyme critical for the synthesis of purines during lymphocyte activation. MPA suppresses DNA synthesis by depleting the guanosine nucleotide pool. In addition to its effects on T cells, MPA inhibits DNA synthesis in fibroblasts and endothelial cells. Also, MPA has been shown to inhibit FGF-stimulated DNA synthesis in smooth muscle cells. By itself, MPA reduces arterial intimal thickening following both mechanical and immune-mediated injury. RPM combined with MPA was the most effective antiproliferative agent tested in our laboratories. The different mechanisms of action appear to combine to produce a very effective antiproliferative effect.

Leflunomide

This is known as LEF. It is a synthetic organic isoxazole derivative that is metabolized to the active form, A77 1726. LEF effectively inhibits T cell proliferation and T cell-dependent antibody synthesis *in vivo*, and successfully treats several animal models of autoimmune diseases in which antibodies play a significant role. While not completely understood, the primary mechanism of action of LEF appears to be blockage of the pyrimidine biosynthetic pathway, thereby inhibiting DNA synthesis. In addition to its ability to inhibit both cellular and humeral responses, LEF also inhibits arterial intimal thickening following alloimmune injury in animal models *in vivo*.

Several other immunosuppressant agents are also effective in preventing the proliferation of nonimmune cells. However, they are not expected to be developed for clinical use, or their future is very uncertain.

What are the potential uses for these agents that inhibit the proliferation of non-immune cells? All cellular inflammatory reactions appear to depend on the interaction of cell surface molecules, cytokines and/or growth factors. The formation of scar tissue, exuberant granulation tissue, keloids and cancers all depend on the stimulation of fibroblasts, endothelial cells and macrophages to produce a structural-vascular complex. Our work has already shown that the three agents listed above are able, *in vivo*, to prevent or reduce arterial intimal thickening associated with various types of injury. The effectiveness of these agents should be tested in other models of inappropriate or exaggerated wound healing.

Nitric oxide

Nitric oxide (NO) is a biological messenger that plays an important role in intracellular communication. NO is generated from the guanidine nitrogens of the amino acid L-arginine. Endothelium-derived NO has a very short life and is quickly converted to the stable end products nitrate and nitrite. The reaction is catalysed by NO synthase; there are at least two constitutively expressed isoforms of this enzyme and one inducible form. One constitutively expressed isoform (endothelial NO synthase, eNOS, type III) produces small amounts of NO and is responsible for changes in vascular tone, and the second isoform (neural NO synthase, nNOS, type I) is found in neural tissue where NO can act as a neurotransmitter. The inducible isoform (induced NO synthase, iNOS, type II) found in macrophages, smooth muscle and other cells can produce large amounts of NO over long periods of time.

NO rapidly reacts with other molecules and passes easily through cell membranes to react with intracellular protein. It has a high affinity for several metals, such as iron and copper, and inhibits the function of several metal-containing proteins. The inhibitory actions of macrophage-derived NO on tumour cell lines include inhibition of DNA synthesis, mitochondrial respiration and the loss of intracellular iron.

NO is postulated to be an endogenously generated immunomodulator. Cytokines (IL-2, INFγ) released by alloreactive T cells, stimulate NO production by graft-infiltrating cells, in particular, macrophages. *In vivo* and *in vitro* studies have shown that excessive NO production during an immune response will inhibit lymphocyte proliferation, acquisition of cytotoxic effector function and antibody synthesis. While antigen-presenting cell/T cell interactions do not appear to be affected by NO, intracellular processing and presentation of antigen by macrophages may be inhibited. NO, induced via the administration of L-arginine, has also been shown to inhibit arterial smooth muscle proliferation following mechanical (balloon catheter) injury. This is believed to be a direct effect on the medial smooth muscle cells: nitric oxide synthase activity is induced in the rat carotid artery within 24 hours of injury and NO suppresses the proliferation of cultured smooth muscle cells.

The production of NO, in large amounts, may inhibit the activation of platelets and neutrophils, the proliferation and activation of T cells, the release of growth factors and the migration and proliferation of smooth muscle cells. NO has been shown to inhibit platelet adherence and aggregation; it also inhibits the adherence of leucocytes, both polymorphonuclear and mononuclear, to endothelium. The impairment of endothelial NO production by hypercholesterolaemia, diabetes mellitus and hypertension appears to play a role in the initiation of atherosclerosis. The administration of L-arginine to hypercholesterolaemic animals results in a significant reduction in atherosclerotic lesions due to inhibition of monocyte–endothelial cell interaction. The administration of L-arginine after balloon angioplasty inhibits myointimal hyperplasia; this effect is antagonized by NO synthase inhibitors.

We found that the administration of L-arginine to rats (a 2.25% solution in tap water) following the creation of random pattern skin flaps resulted in a 9% increase in flap survival over animals receiving no treatment. When rats were given a NO antagonist, flap survival fell almost 2% from the survival of flaps from untreated rats. The increased survival of the flaps on rats that had received L-arginine was attributed to vasodilation induced by nitric oxide; thus, arterial vasospasm was reduced preserving perfusion in the distal aspects of the random pattern flaps. L-Arginine was also administered to rats receiving growth factors. In combination, L-arginine and growth factors, and in particular TGF-β, significantly increased flap survival. This approach to augmenting nitric oxide levels following or prior to wounding may have application in several clinical situations. In particular, L-arginine could be administered prior to surgery to animals that may be prone to poor wound healing, such as diabetics, burn patients and patients with severely infected wounds.

CONCLUSIONS

Wound healing can be enhanced by simple, inexpensive and readily available means. Preoperative evaluation should identify impediments to healing, such as malnutrition, anaemia, hyperglycaemia and steroid use and allow correction prior to surgery. Intraoperatively, the surgeon should apply proper and gentle technique, appropriate antibiotic use and prevention of vasoconstriction by maintaining plasma volume and body temperature. Postoperatively, the clinician should focus on the prevention of vasoconstriction through pain relief, warming, and maintenance of plasma volume as well as the maintenance of normoglycaemia. In chronic non-healing wounds, the institution of growth factor and/or nitric oxide therapy may stimulate more rapid healing.

REFERENCES AND FURTHER READING

Carlson MA (1997) Acute wound failure. *Surgical Clinics of North America* **77**, 607–636

Hunt TK and Williams Hopf H (1997) Wound healing and wound infection. *Surgical Clinics of North America* **77**, 587–606

Pascoe JR (1992) Wound healing. In: *Atlas of Small Animal Surgery*, ed. IMG Gourley and CR Gregory, pp.1.2–1.11. Gower Medical Publishing, New York

Witte MB and Barbul A (1997) General principles of wound healing. *Surgical Clinics of North America* **77**, 509–528

CHAPTER FOUR

Wound Closure Options and Decision Making

Jamie R. Bellah and John M. Williams

INTRODUCTION

There are many different types of wound encountered in veterinary practice, e.g. lacerations, degloving wounds (either anatomical or physiological), wounds secondary to crushing or shearing injuries, gunshot wounds and surgical wounds. No one method can be applied for their management. One of the first questions a veterinary surgeon must answer when faced with a traumatic wound is whether or not the wound is amenable to immediate closure. If the answer is no, then appropriate open wound management must be instituted, and a decision made regarding the appropriate timing of subsequent wound closure. Finally, the veterinary surgeon must decide on an acceptable, or optimal, method of wound reconstruction. This chapter sets out the chronological priorities of wound management and the factors that must be considered in instituting appropriate wound therapy. Specific details of many procedures are covered in later chapters.

SYSTEMIC EVALUATION AND PAIN MANAGEMENT

When the patient first presents it is imperative to assess the magnitude of injury completely. Animals suffering from traumatic wounds frequently have concomitant injury to other organ systems. Systemic injury must be recognized and treated appropriately prior to implementing specific therapy for the more obvious cutaneous wounds (see Figures 1.2 and 1.3). Haemorrhage, hypovolaemia, urinary tract trauma, thoracic and pulmonary injury, orthopaedic injury and head trauma are all common in animals presenting with traumatic open wounds, depending upon the aetiology of the injury.

Once the animal is stabilized it is appropriate to consider sedation, analgesia or general anaesthesia depending on the condition of the patient and the status of the wound. Pain relief is important for animal welfare and also helps minimize the risk of the patient becoming catabolic, with its adverse effects on wound healing and increased risk of nosocomial infection. Careful selection of analgesics also aids in the choice of anaesthetic regimen.

Analgesic agents include the opioids, non-steroidal anti-inflammatory drugs (NSAIDs) and local anaesthetics (Figure 4.1). Opioids are the cornerstone of analgesic regimens in the trauma patient despite their potential side effects of respiratory depression, bradycardia, altered mental state and vomiting. In general, patients in pain are less likely to exhibit these side effects. NSAIDs are valuable as analgesics but must be administered with care in traumatized patients due to their potential adverse effect on renal and gastrointestinal function. Newer NSAIDs such as carprofen and meloxicam have minimal effects in this area. Local and regional anaesthetic techniques have the advantage of diminished systemic effects, whilst providing total local analgesia. Either lignocaine (lidocaine, USA) or the longer acting bupivicaine can be used. It is important to remember that cavalier use of local anaesthetic agents can lead to systemic toxicity. Therefore, total tolerable doses should be calculated prior to administration. Detailed descriptions of these techniques are found in many texts including the *BSAVA Manual of Small Animal Anaesthesia and Analgesia*.

Fractious patients, in pain, frequently require sedation or general anaesthesia prior to thorough evaluation of the wound. Sedatives can be used alone or in combination with analgesics, either solely to aid in calming and reducing pain in the trauma patient or as a premedicant prior to proposed general anaesthesia. Of the three major groups of sedatives (phenothiazines, α_2 agonists, benzodiazepines), α_2 agonists are not recommended in trauma patients due to their potentially profound depression of the cardiovascular and respiratory systems. A detailed discussion of sedative and anaesthetic protocols for the traumatized patient is outside the scope of this manual and the reader is referred to the *BSAVA Manual of Canine and Feline Emergency and Critical Care* and the *BSAVA Manual of Small Animal Anaesthesia and Analgesia*.

EVALUATING THE WOUND: TO CLOSE OR NOT TO CLOSE?

Wounds are often complicated by contaminating bacteria and foreign debris, or may be infected secondarily

Drug	Side effects	Efficacy	Dose	Route	Duration of action	Comments
Buprenorphine (Opioid; partial agonist)	Respiratory depression, bradycardia, altered mental state, vomiting	Slow onset. Good for 'moderate' degree of pain. Dose 'plateau' means that increase in dosage is not beneficial	Cats, dogs: 0.006–0.02 mg/kg	i.v., i.m. or s.c.	3–8 hours	Licensed for use in dogs (Schedule 3 Controlled Drug in the UK)
Butorphanol (Opioid; agonist/antagonist)	Respiratory depression, bradycardia, altered mental state, vomiting	Questionable efficacy as sole analgesic agent	Cats: 0.2–0.8 mg/kg; Dogs: 0.2–0.5 mg/kg	i.m. or s.c.	Short acting. Dogs: Up to 3 hours. Cats: 2–4 hours	Licensed for dogs and cats (Schedule 3 Controlled Drug in the UK)
Morphine (Opioid; agonist)	Respiratory depression, bradycardia, altered mental state, vomiting	Time of onset = 15 min. Powerful analgesia	Cats: 0.1–0.4 mg/kg; Dogs: 0.2–1.0 mg/kg	s.c., i.m. or slow i.v. (may be hypotensive)	Variable, depends on degree of pain 1–4 hours	Non-licensed for use in dogs and cats (Schedule 2 Controlled Drug in the UK)
Pethidine (meperidine, USA) (Opioid; agonist)	Respiratory depression, minimal bradycardia, altered mental state, vomiting, histamine release if given i.v.	Rapid onset. Short duration	Cats, dogs: 2–5 mg/kg	i.m.	2 hours (max)	Licensed for use in dogs (Schedule 2 Controlled Drug in the UK)
Oxymorphone (Opioid; agonist)	Respiratory depression, bradycardia, vomiting. Less of an altered mental state induced in cats compared to other drugs		Cats: 0.02–0.1 mg/kg; Dogs: 0.05–0.2 mg/kg	i.v., i.m. or s.c.	2–6 hours	Licensed for use in dogs in the USA
Methadone (Opioid; agonist)	Respiratory depression, bradycardia, altered mental state, vomiting	Poor analgesic effect. Minimal practical value	Cats, dogs: 0.25 mg/kg	i.m.	Variable	Non-licensed for use in dogs and cats (Schedule 2 Controlled Drug in the UK)
Fentanyl (Opioid; agonist)	Profound respiratory depression, profound bradycardia, altered mental state, vomiting	Rapid onset (2–7 min). Very potent analgesic BUT apnoea may occur – best reserved for intraoperative balanced anaesthesia	Cats, dogs: 2–5 µg/kg	i.v.	Short 15–20 min	Non-licensed for use in dogs and cats (Schedule 2 Controlled Drug in the UK)
Fentanyl transdermal patch (Opioid; agonist)	Respiratory depression, bradycardia, altered mental state, vomiting. Contraindicated in hepatic disease	Slow onset 12–24 hours. Continuous delivery. Can partially cover delivery membrane for cats and small dogs	Cats, dogs: 2–4 µg/kg/h	Transdermal. Four sizes of patch: 25, 50, 75 and 100 µg/h	72 hours	Non-licensed for use in dogs and cats (Schedule 2 Controlled Drug in the UK)
Carprofen (NSAID)	GI irritation and ulceration, renal papillary necrosis. Do not use in dehydrated or hypovolaemic cases. Do not use with corticosteroid	Minimal side effects but DO NOT give within 24 hours of other NSAIDs	Cats, dogs: 4 mg/kg	i.m., s.c. or i.v.	Lasts up to 24 hours	Licensed for dogs and cats

Figure 4.1: Common analgesics.

as wound contamination progresses into wound infection. It is important to assess the host's natural defence mechanisms, to estimate the number and virulence of bacteria that have contaminated the wound, and to consider the time interval and the care provided to the wound since injury.

The question of whether to close, and when to close, any cutaneous wound must be asked continually from the moment of initial wound inspection and throughout any subsequent phases of open wound management. There are no hard and fast rules as each wound is different; however, if there is any doubt, especially with regard to the level of contamination and infection, the wound should not be closed. Rather, appropriate open wound management should be instituted (see Chapter 5 for further details) until such time as wound closure is possible. Closing a wound that is contaminated can have disastrous consequences for both the wound and the patient. This is a lesson which, unfortunately, has been learned, and forgotten, in many major wars of the twentieth century. It is now fully accepted, in both human medical and veterinary wound care, that open management is an appropriate and often essential step in optimal wound care.

Individual wounds vary depending on their aetiology and the degree and duration of contamination resulting from the trauma. The type of wound (abrasion, avulsion, incision, laceration, puncture, or crushing injury) is indicative of the severity of injury and the potential for ischaemia, contamination and the type of bacterial flora that may contribute to eventual wound infection. The two most important factors in determining the suitability of any wound for closure are:

- The degree of wound contamination
- The extent of wound ischaemia.

Level of contamination

Wounds are classified as: clean; clean–contaminated; contaminated; or dirty/infected.

Clean wounds

These are made under sterile conditions without invasion of gastrointestinal, respiratory, genitourinary or oropharyngeal cavities. By definition, clean wounds are limited to surgical procedures.

Clean–contaminated wounds

These have minimal contamination, which is readily removed or reduced to a biologically insignificant level. Surgical wounds involving the gastrointestinal, respiratory, genitourinary or oropharyngeal cavities are considered clean–contaminated. Traumatic wounds should not be considered clean–contaminated at the time of initial presentation, but may be converted to a clean–contaminated state through lavage and debridement.

Contaminated wounds

These have heavy contamination, often associated with foreign material within the wound. Surgical procedures with a major break in aseptic technique, such as spillage of gastrointestinal contents, or acutely presented traumatic wounds are considered contaminated.

Dirty wounds

These are associated with wound infection, as would be expected from a perforated viscus or in an old traumatic wound with a septic purulent exudate.

It is apparent that, by definition, traumatic open wounds are always contaminated or dirty at the time of presentation. Also, by definition, traumatic open wounds can never be converted into a clean state. Wound closure should be considered when, and only when, the wound has been converted from a contaminated or dirty state into a clean–contaminated state through lavage and debridement.

Extent of wound ischaemia

Vascular injury that results in tissue ischaemia predisposes to wound infection. The vascular damage resulting from crush injuries and high-velocity gunshot wounds extends beyond the grossly identifiable boundaries of the wound. Tissue viability is often difficult to discern accurately at the time of the injury, and repeated debridement is frequently required. If in doubt as to the viability of tissues surrounding the wound, it is best to institute open wound management (see Chapter 5). The wound is assessed, lavaged and debrided on a daily or twice-daily basis until ongoing tissue necrosis is controlled. Layered debridement of the wound is generally preferred. However, if structures surrounding the wound are non-vital, and if the wound is located anatomically in an area with ample soft tissue, *en bloc* debridement is carried out.

In assessing the effects of wound ischaemia, it is also important to consider vascular damage to deeper, critical tissues, such as bone. Open fractures associated with extensive soft tissue loss are prone to the development of osteomyelitis, delayed healing and non-union. Early reconstruction of the wound with vascularized tissue is indicated in the management of such wounds. Identification of non-viable tissue and adequate debridement are still essential, but prolonged periods of open wound management should be avoided. Most wounds can be converted from a contaminated or dirty state into a clean–contaminated state, with no ongoing tissue necrosis, within 72 hours of injury if aggressive and appropriate open wound management is employed.

TIMING OF WOUND CLOSURE

Wounds of the integument may be treated by primary closure, delayed primary closure or secondary closure, or may be left to heal by second intention (Figure 4.2).

Closure option	Wound type	Technique
Primary closure	Clean	Immediate closure without tension May require grafting or appropriate flap technique
Delayed primary closure	Clean-contaminated or contaminated, questionable tissue viability, oedema, skin tension likely	Lavage and debridement of open wound Appropriate dressing used Closure performed 2-3 days after wounding May require grafting or appropriate flap technique
Secondary closure	Contaminated or dirty	Lavage and debridement of open wound Appropriate dressing used Closure carried out 5-7 days after wounding May require grafting or appropriate flap technique
Second intention healing	Wound unsuitable for closure technique, large skin deficits, extensive contamination and devitalization	Lavage and debridement of open wound Appropriate dressing used Allowed to heal by granulation, contraction and epithelialization

Figure 4.2: Closure options and wound type.

Primary closure

This is performed immediately after presentation, following acute lavage and debridement of the wound. Closure of the wound leaves little risk of infection, with the expectation that normal wound healing will occur. Primary closure should only be performed on clean or clean-contaminated wounds with little potential for ischaemic injury (e.g. recent sharp lacerations).

Delayed primary closure

This is done 3-5 days after the wound occurs. This delay allows elimination of exudate and/or contamination that might cause complications of the normal wound healing process, as well as identification and debridement of non-viable tissues. By definition, delayed primary closure is performed prior to the appearance of granulation tissue within the wound.

Secondary closure

This is done following open wound treatment that extends beyond 5 days, allowing complete debridement and management of an infected wound before closure. By definition, secondary closure is performed after the appearance of granulation tissue in the wound.

Second intention healing

This is defined as wound healing by granulation, contraction and re-epithelialization. Second intention healing is generally reserved for wounds located in areas with abundant surrounding skin, or for smaller wounds located on the extremities.

Factors determining timing of wound closure

As indicated above, the most critical factors in determining how quickly the wound can be closed include the level of wound contamination (must be clean-contaminated) and the viability of tissues surrounding the wound (must be free of ongoing tissue necrosis). However, not all surgeons elect to close or reconstruct wounds at the earliest opportunity. In many instances, it may be more economical to allow wounds to heal by second intention. Early wound reconstruction is advised, however, if:

- Vital structures are exposed
- Tissue reconstruction is needed for structural support
- Wounds are located over the flexor surface of a joint, where prolonged open wound management may favour the development of contracture and joint dysfunction.

In deciding whether or not to close a wound it is important to take into account the function of the surrounding tissue. In some cases it is wholly inappropriate to allow a wound to close by contraction and epithelialization. Wound contraction and epithelialization may result in an inability to extend a joint if a large wound over the flexor surface is allowed to heal by second intention (Figure 4.3). This complication is termed wound contracture. In contracture, the inelastic scar tissue produced leads to contraction, preventing complete extension of the limb. Scar tissue will also restrict the gliding motion of tendons and, secondarily, limit flexion of joints such as the carpus.

Wound contraction or tension from reconstruction may also interfere with the function of eyelids or lips. Therefore, surgical restoration of skin coverage in these areas must maintain function. Preservation of vital weight-bearing tissues such as footpads is also important in wound reconstruction after tumour removal or traumatic injury involving the paws.

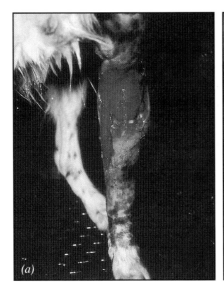

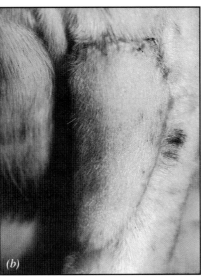

Figure 4.3: (a) *Wound over the flexor surface of the elbow in a mixed breed dog. Allowing such a wound to heal by second intention would result in severe reduction of joint function. This wound was managed by using a tubed pedicle flap.* (b) *A fully functional elbow following resection of the pedicle tube.*

Finally, function may be compromised by the wounding incident itself. Figure 4.4 shows a Sheltie that had sustained a degloving injury to its tail immediately prior to presentation. Careful examination revealed that the dorsal two thirds of the anal sphincter had avulsed with the skin and the right perineal diaphragm was disrupted. The wound was classified as contaminated. After stabilization of the dog, the wound was clipped, prepared and thoroughly lavaged, and primary closure was achieved. The tail was amputated, the right perineal diaphragm was repaired and the skin was apposed in two layers to the rectal wall and mucosa and anal sphincter remnant. The dog's quality of life was salvaged, though normal faecal continence could not be restored.

THE ROLE OF SYSTEMIC ANTIBIOTICS

The role of antibiotics in wound management is controversial. Systemic antibiotics prevent bacterial mul-

tiplication for up to 3 hours, with a maximal effect at around 1 hour. It is, therefore, better to have high circulating levels of antibiotics at the time of the trauma/contaminating incident than afterwards. This obviously is not clinically realistic, except in the instance of surgically induced wounds.

If systemic antibiotics are to be used, they should be directed against the most likely contaminants, usually coagulase-positive staphylococci, *Escherichia coli* or *Pasteurella* sp., depending upon the aetiology of the wound. In the case of established wound infection, the selection of a specific antibiotic should be based on culture and sensitivity results. Antibiotics are not a substitute for wound lavage and debridement and should only be used in conjunction with these procedures.

There is little controversy regarding the need for systemic antibiotics in the management of clinically infected wounds. In this instance, antibiotics are used therapeutically to treat an established infection. Invasive bacterial infection in the wound is generally associated with systemic signs of illness, such as fever,

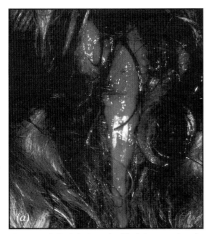

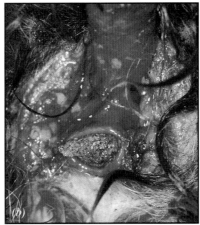

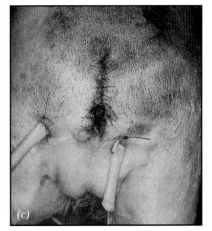

Figure 4.4: (a) *A male Sheltie sustained a complete tail degloving injury following a road traffic accident. The dog was presented immediately after the injury.* (b) *Elevation of the degloved tail revealed that the dorsal two thirds of the anal sphincter was missing and the right perineal diaphragm was torn.* (c) *Reconstruction was carried out following thorough lavage and tail amputation. The right perineal diaphragm was repaired and a two-layer apposition of the surrounding skin was made to the rectal wall and mucosa and the ventral anal sphincter remnant.*

malaise and inappetance. Complete blood counts frequently reveal varying degrees of neutrophilia and left shift associated with significant wound infection. Excessive inflammatory reaction at the wound, characterized by severe soft tissue swelling, erythema, pain and purulent discharge is also indicative of wound infection.

The role of systemic antibiotics for the management of contaminated wounds is much less clear. In the absence of established wound infection the use of antibiotics is prophylactic. In other words, antibiotics are used to decrease the risk or incidence of wound infection. The use of prophylactic antibiotics in non-infected open wounds, however, may not reduce the actual incidence of wound infection because of the ongoing exposure of the wound to new hospital contaminants. In the instance of contaminated wounds treated open, systemic antibiotics may, in fact, encourage the establishment of nosocomial or antibiotic-resistant infections. Therefore, contaminated wounds are probably best managed through judicious debridement and lavage, with antibiotic use reserved for instances of established or developing wound infection. It should also be remembered that, following the appearance of healthy granulation tissue in the wound, the risk of wound infection is quite low.

WOUND CLOSURE TECHNIQUES

Once the decision has been made to close a wound, the surgeon must decide on the optimal method of wound closure or reconstruction. Regardless of the specific reconstructive technique used, it is essential to adhere to Halstead's principles of surgery (see Figure 1.1). Tissues must be handled gently to prevent further vascular injury and an increased inflammatory response. Control of haemorrhage reduces the risk of systemic complications secondary to hypovolaemia, reduces the risk of postoperative infection, and diminishes the incidence of haematoma and seroma formation. Accurate identification of tissue layers and precise apposition of tissues reduce the incidence of dehiscence and improve the quality and cosmetic result of the reconstruction. All wound edges, following surgical debridement, should be vertical, to allow true apposition with minimal scar formation. Dead space is common following wound reconstruction and should be managed by suture apposition of deep tissue layers or application of passive or active drains.

One of the cardinal rules of wound reconstruction is to avoid excessive wound tension. Wounds with adequate elastic surrounding skin can be closed using direct skin mobilization. Appositional suturing techniques can be used to minimize tension on the wound. Placement of skin sutures is important so that optimal healing will occur; sutures should be placed some 5 mm from wound edges and spaced at intervals of 5 mm so that tension is spread evenly and there is minimal interference with local blood supply. Sutures should not be tied too tightly as, in addition to causing discomfort, they will disrupt local blood supply and lead to delayed healing. Figures 4.5 and 4.6 show optimal placement; note the slight wound eversion on needle placement which will flatten out as the wound heals. Care must be taken when using tension relieving sutures as it is all too easy to overtighten these, especially mattress sutures where large areas of skin can potentially become devitalized.

Wound contraction can be noted in healing open wounds in 5-9 days, and results in a centripetal reduction in the size of the wound. The process of wound contraction stops when wound margins contact each other or when tension from the skin adjacent to the wound is equal to, or greater than, the contractile forces generated by myofibroblasts within the granulation tissue. In dogs and cats, wound

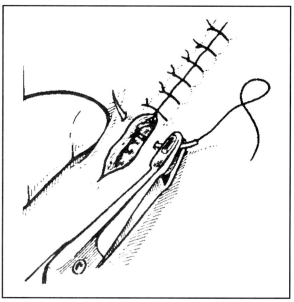

Figure 4.5: *Simple interrupted sutures placed with slight eversion of the wound edges. The wound edge can be everted using fine tissue forceps, skin hooks or a thumb.*

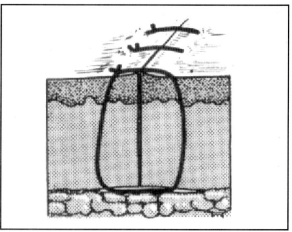

Figure 4.6: *Simple interrupted sutures taking in a greater amount of the deep part of the dermis. This helps maintain direct wound apposition.*

contraction is more rapid on the trunk than the extremities because of the larger amount of skin available and its inherent elasticity.

Wound contraction is facilitated by:

- A moist wound bed
- Adequate debridement
- Control of wound infection.

Inadequate debridement is the most common reason for delayed wound healing and persistent wound infection. Wound contraction is delayed by:

- Wound infection
- Desiccation
- Exposed bone
- Exuberant granulation tissue.

The normal process of wound contraction can be facilitated by:

- Presuturing lesions prior to excision
- Placement of tension sutures
- Using skin stretching devices across open wounds.

Closure of large trunk wounds, or smaller wounds of the extremities, may be difficult without excessive tension. The elastic properties of skin can be used to advantage in these situations. Presuturing of wounds, by the placement of several mattress sutures adjacent to the area of excision, can be used to mobilize skin for subsequent wound reconstruction in planned excisions. In traumatic wounds, intradermal tension sutures can be placed along the wound edges. The continuous intradermal suture is tightened on a daily basis, facilitating contraction of the wound margins. This process of 'enhanced contraction' will greatly reduce the length of time required to achieve closure of large cutaneous deficits.

Managing large tissue deficits

If simple tension relieving techniques appear to place undue tension on the wound, more advanced reconstructive techniques, such as subdermal plexus flaps, axial pattern skin flaps or free skin grafts, should be considered. Once debridement and preparation are complete, surgical reconstruction is planned. Reconstructive techniques help to achieve early coverage of vital structures and promote an early return to function. The following sections introduce various reconstructive techniques used for wound closure; these will be discussed in greater depth in later chapters.

Axial pattern skin flaps

Axial pattern flap circulation depends on preserving a direct cutaneous artery at the flap's base. The flap will survive based only on the vascular attachment. These flaps can be made much longer than subdermal plexus flaps; therefore, their utility is greater and their ability to manage large defects of the extremities or the trunk by immediate closure is an advantage. In addition, axial flaps provide full thickness skin and can be combined in some regions with muscle, resulting in musculocutaneous composite flaps. The major disadvantage of axial flaps is that flap designs are restricted to the sites with an extensive direct cutaneous artery. (See Chapter 8 for further details.)

Skin grafts

Free skin grafts may be of split or full thickness with little or full hair growth, respectively. They may be applied immediately to sterile wound beds with good blood supply, such as regions of the face or on muscular surfaces, or to mature granulation tissue. Variations of free skin grafts include sieve, punch, meshed and strip grafts. (See Chapter 9 for more details.)

Pedicled muscle flaps

These flaps are used to provide vascularized soft tissue coverage of vital structures and for padding of bony prominences such as the elbow. For example, cranial sartorius muscle flaps are used to close abdominal wall defects or to cover exposed bone after disarticulated rear limb amputations. Musculocutaneous flaps supplied by the thoracodorsal artery and vein, including cutaneous trunci and a portion of the latissimus dorsi muscle, can be used to cover defects involving the elbow in dogs or cats (Figure 4.7). Pedicled muscle

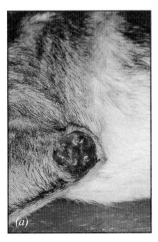
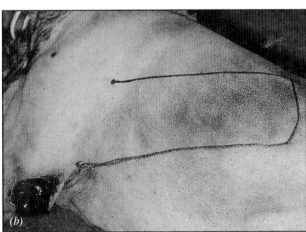

Figure 4.7: (a) A large, raised open wound lateral and caudal in the region of the elbow that was suspected to be an infected hygroma. The wound did not respond to antimicrobial treatment and biopsy revealed an anaplastic sarcoma. (b) En bloc *tumour excision was performed, followed by reconstruction using a thoracodorsal axial pattern flap together with the underlying latissimus dorsi muscle. The margins of the flap have been outlined.*

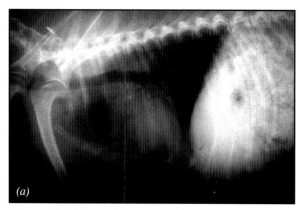 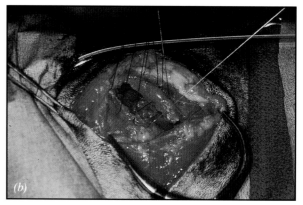

Figure 4.8: (a) *Lateral thoracic radiograph of a mixed breed dog with bite wounds over the thoracic cavity. This view and the ventrodorsal view showed no detectable abnormal findings when taken 2 hours after the injury.* (b) *Surgical exploration of the bite wounds revealed intercostal lacerations exposing the diaphragm and pleural cavity. This wound required aggressive debridement, thorough lavage and chest drain insertion before closure.*

flaps are also useful for covering exposed bone or joints after traumatic exposure with skin loss. (See Chapter 10 for more details.)

Microvascular free tissue transfer

Free flap transfer using microvascular anastomosis to restore circulation after temporary interruption of blood supply provides a technically difficult but very useful method of covering difficult architectural defects by primary repair. Cutaneous, musculocutaneous and muscle flaps can be harvested from distant sites, moved directly to recipient areas, and sutured in place after vascular anastomosis. (See Chapter 11 for further details.)

PRACTICAL APPLICATIONS

The following case examples demonstrate the practical application of various options for wound management.

Bite wounds

Bite wounds are very common injuries in small animals. Most are managed routinely by lavage, debridement, temporary drainage and wound closure. Bite wounds that occur over body cavities are often serious; although the skin puncture wounds are very small, there may be soft tissue and, occasionally, orthopaedic damage beneath (see Figures 12.12 and 12.13). Bite wounds result in a combination of crushing and lacerating injury to tissue, with significant vascular disruption and inoculation of oral flora. Abdominal wall hernia or vascular injury to splanchnic and gastrointestinal viscera may occur with bites over the abdominal cavity. Pleurocutaneous fistulae and diaphragmatic lacerations can occur when the thoracic cavity is involved.

Animals with bite wounds that occur over body cavities should be examined carefully for evidence of shock or visceral injury. In addition to physical examination, radiographs of the thorax and abdomen should be obtained to assess potential injury to deeper structures. Pleural or peritoneal air and fluid, rib fracture, diaphragmatic hernia, and sternal or vertebral subluxation or fracture may be identified. It must be remembered that radiographs made soon after the traumatic event may not reveal internal injuries (Figure 4.8a).

Once the patient is stabilized, and if concomitant injuries do not preclude anaesthesia and surgery, the bite wounds should be explored to identify the extent of damage under the skin. If the wound penetrates a body cavity the dissection is extended to explore the cavity, as needed, to assess intra-abdominal or intrathoracic injury. Thoracic bite wounds should be explored with the anticipation of entering the pleural space (Figure 4.8b). Intercostal lacerations are common and may or may not result in dramatic pneumothorax. When abdominal bite wounds are explored and traumatic herniation is evident, the entire abdomen must be explored for visceral damage. Thorough lavage with isotonic isothermic fluid is indicated to dilute contamination. Free blood clots within body cavities are removed as they provide a nidus for bacterial growth, isolated from host defence mechanisms. Blood clots attached to damaged viscera, such as liver or splenic fractures and pulmonary lacerations, should be left in place so that haemorrhage or air leakage is not re-started. Appropriate drainage of the pleural space via tube thoracostomy is usually required for 24–48 hours. Depending on the degree of abdominal contamination, and following debridement of all wounds, the peritoneal cavity may be closed primarily or open peritoneal drainage may be undertaken.

Extremity wounds

Allowing wounds to heal, at least in part, by second intention can make secondary closure by local methods easier to perform and may help reduce tension across a wound (Figure 4.9). Wounds of the extremi-

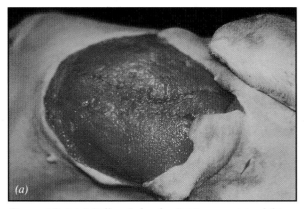 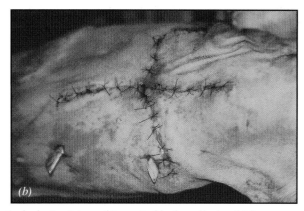

Figure 4.9: (a) A Yellow Labrador Retriever sustained this anatomic degloving injury of its ventral body wall when hit by a car. Partial closure was performed after the initial lavage and debridement. (b) Secondary closure by local skin mobilization using walking sutures was achieved 3 weeks after the original injury. Granulation tissue was mature and wound contraction had begun to narrow the diameter of the wound.

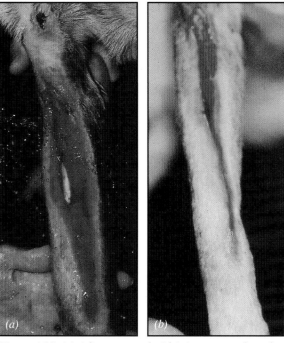

Figure 4.10: (a) A linear wound with injury to muscle and exposed bone in a mixed breed dog hit by a car. (b) Initial surgical debridement was followed by wet-to-dry wound dressings. Granulation tissue production, wound contraction and re-epithelialization resulted in nearly complete resolution of the wound within 4 weeks.

Wounds without exposure of vital structures, but that have severe contamination or the presence of wound infection, benefit from open wound management prior to definitive closure. Repeated debridement to remove debris, devitalized tissue or bone fragments, and open wound management to drain exudate from the wound, are essential to prepare for delayed primary closure or reconstruction (Figure 4.11).

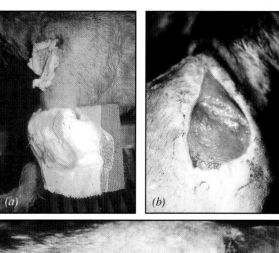

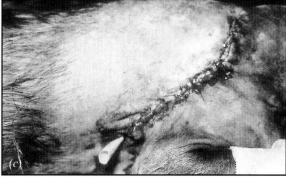

Figure 4.11: A male Yorkshire Terrier sustained severe injuries to both shoulders secondary to a dog fight. Skin, subcutaneous tissue, muscle and scapular injury occurred. Devitalized tissue including scapular bone fragments were debrided from both shoulders. (a) Wet-to-dry dressings were used, shown here on the left shoulder. (b) Mature granulation tissue is shown in the right shoulder. (c) Both shoulder wounds were subsequently closed over Penrose drains (right shoulder illustrated).

ties that are oriented parallel to the limb will heal by second intention with a narrow linear scar (Figure 4.10). Early after the trauma such a wound may appear wide and difficult to repair primarily, but swelling often makes the tissue defect appear wider than it actually is. Once swelling subsides, in 3–5 days, a definitive closure can be planned. Attempts to close extremity wounds early after trauma can result in circumferential tension and obstruction of lymphatic and venous return from the distal regions of the limbs. In the absence of exposed vital structures, it is appropriate to consider delaying wound closure until swelling subsides.

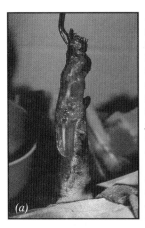

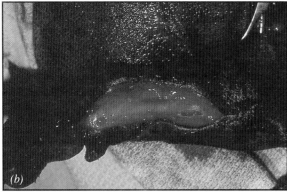

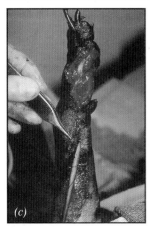

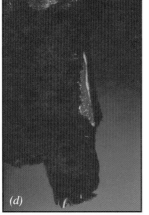

Figure 4.12: (a) A Toy Poodle sustained a shearing injury to the antebrachium and carpus, resulting in extensor tendon injury and exposed radiocarpal and intercarpal joints. (b,c) After debridement, lavage and stabilization of the radiocarpal joint, a releasing incision was made on the contralateral side of the antebrachium and a 'bipedical flap' was advanced to cover the exposed portion of the carpus and implants. (d) The releasing incision wound healed readily by second intention.

Vital structures are sometimes exposed in traumatic wounds (Figure 4.12a). Debridement and early coverage with vascularized tissue is indicated to protect these vital structures from desiccation and additional trauma. If there is insufficient local tissue to cover the vital structures easily, mobilization of muscle or skin flaps may be performed. A releasing incision, parallel to the long axis of the limb, is one method of mobilizing local skin on the extremity to allow coverage of open joint surfaces or exposed tendons (Figure 4.12b,c). The wound created by the releasing incision forms granulation tissue readily and heals quickly (Figure 4.12d).

Muscle flaps in the vicinity of an injury can also be mobilized and rotated on a vascular pedicle to provide coverage of exposed joint surfaces, depending on the joint involved. Such vascularized tissue provides a barrier to infection between exposed vital structures and the environment, allows access for cellular and humoral immune mechanisms to access the wound, and provides a good surface for the formation of granulation tissue.

Wounds associated with orthopaedic injury

Joint trauma

Injuries associated with joint trauma should be debrided carefully of debris, clots and cartilage fragments and lavaged thoroughly. Large fragments that have soft tissue attachment may be rigidly stabilized and, where possible, the surrounding ligaments and joint capsule sutured using fine monofilament absorbable suture material. The joint should be covered by well vascularized soft tissue, if possible, and stabilized. Stabilization may be accomplished using external co-aptation (e.g. a half cast that can be changed daily) or by use of external or ring fixators to stabilize the articulation more rigidly while granulation tissue is produced within the wound (Figure 4.13). Stabilization is especially important if the joint surface cannot be covered with vascularized tissue.

Fractures

Wounds associated with orthopaedic injury are sufficiently painful that stabilization of the injury by internal or external fixation is required to decrease discomfort. Additionally, stabilization facilitates wound healing by reparative tissues. Figure 4.14a is a lateral thoracic radiograph of a dog with a sternal fracture and an associated pleurocutaneous fistula. One of the major reasons for exploring this wound (Figure 4.14b), in addition to determining the extent of subcutaneous tissue and chest wall damage under the skin, was to alleviate the pain associated with sternal luxation and instability. Similar benefits are noted with complicated fractures of the extremities or mandible.

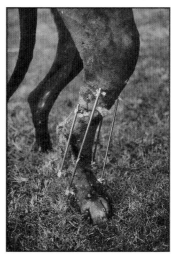

Figure 4.13: A transarticular external fixator has been used to stabilize an open wound involving the tibiotarsal joint in a Great Dane. This allowed for daily wound care and protection of reparative granulation tissue.

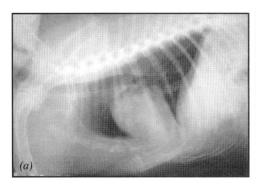
(a)

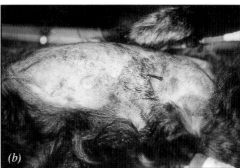
(b)

*Figure 4.14:
(a) Lateral thoracic
radiograph showing
severe sternal fracture
displacement. (b) The
sternal fracture
displacement which had
resulted from a dog bite
injury. The heart beat
was easily palpable
through the wound.*

Atypical wounds

Wounds that appear to be traumatic or associated with foreign bodies are sometimes actually second-ary to atypical infection or neoplasia. Such wounds typically do not respond completely to conventional open wound management. Figures 4.7, 4.15 and 4.16 demonstrate infected wounds that did not respond to appropriate wound care because of anaplastic sar-coma, pithiosis, and phycomycosis, respectively. Atypical mycobacterial infection can also produce chronic non-healing wounds or draining tracts (Fig-ure 4.17). Surgical biopsy is indicated for prolifera-tive or ulcerative wounds that do not respond appropriately to open wound management.

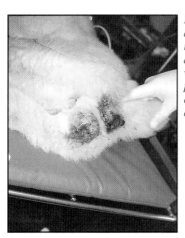

*Figure 4.15: A
draining vulvar mass,
non-responsive to
antimicrobial therapy,
was diagnosed as
pithiosis by biopsy and
culture in this 4-year-
old female Chow Chow.*

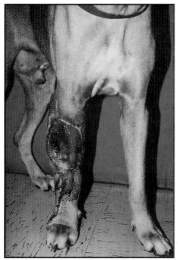

*Figure 4.16: A chronic
non-responsive
proliferative wound
secondary to a
cutaneous fungal
infection, and
complicated by self-
trauma is present in
this Rhodesian
Ridgeback.*

Courtesy of Dr Gary Ellison.

Proliferative granulomatous lesions secondary to phycomycosis, pithiosis and mycobacterial infection are diagnosed only by culture of wound tissue. Silver stains for fungal organisms or acid-fast stains for myco-bacterial organisms can reveal the organisms on tissue imprints made for cytological examination. Complete surgical debridement may be possible depending on the location of the wound; however, recurrence is common. Mycobacterial infection often responds to macrolide or tetracyline antimicrobial therapy, whereas pithiosis and phycomycosis tend to recur locally. *Pithium* spreads locally and systemically via lymphatic channels and infection can mimic neoplastic disease.

Neoplastic disease that is secondarily infected is diagnosed by biopsy; prognosis depends on the ability to obtain surgical tumour-free margins and the indi-vidual tumour's anticipated clinical behaviour, and stage of disease (see Chapter 1).

Figure 4.18 shows the footpad of a large mixed breed dog examined for a chronic draining footpad wound that the owners thought had occurred second-ary to a penetrating foreign body. Antimicrobial treat-ment and general wound care had resulted in no improvement. Incisional biopsy revealed the firm mass to be a sweat gland carcinoma. *En bloc* excision using frozen sections to detect margins resulted in salvage of as much metacarpal pad as possible and normal

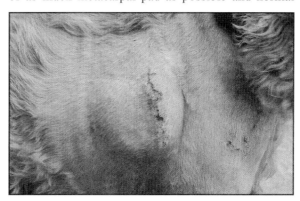

*Figure 4.17: A Cocker Spaniel sustained bite wounds that
were initially treated by surgical debridement and closure
over a Penrose drain. Swelling and drainage occurred within
10 days. The mass was re-excised but again recurred. A third
excision was examined histopathologically and acid-fast
organisms were seen. A culture was not performed, but 3
months of erythromycin resulted in cessation of clinical
signs, and atypical mycobacterial infection was suspected.*

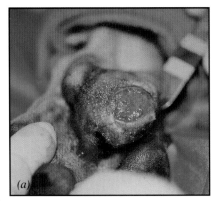 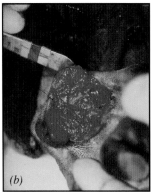 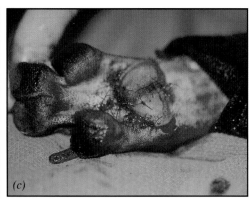

Figure 4.18: (a) A large mixed breed dog was examined because of a draining tract from a carpal footpad thought to originate *from stepping on a foreign body. Biopsy revealed sweat gland carcinoma. (b) Frozen sections were obtained at surgery until clean surgical margins were detected to allow conservation of as much footpad tissue as possible. (c) Releasing incisions abaxial to the footpad remnants allowed sufficient mobilization to appose the footpad components, reforming a smaller but adequate carpal pad. A spoon splint was used for 21 days to protect the footpad incision.*

weight-bearing was achieved in the long term.

Squamous cell carcinomas frequently present as ulcer-like lesions on the skin or oral cavity or other mucocutaneous junctions; failure to heal or respond to medical therapy indicates that a biopsy is required.

FURTHER READING

Harari J (1993) *Surgical Complications and Wound Healing in the Small Animal Practice.* WB Saunders, Philadelphia

Swaim S and Henderson R (1997) *Small Animal Wound Management.* Williams and Wilkins, Baltimore

CHAPTER FIVE

Open Wound Management

John M. Williams

EVALUATION OF THE WOUND

When evaluating a wound it is essential to assess the patient's vital parameters and deal with any concurrent injuries, e.g. orthopaedic injuries, thoracic injuries. With any wound a thorough understanding of the principles of wound healing and bacteriology is essential. Wounds can be classified in a number of ways, but from the standpoint of treatment there are essentially only two types of wound: those that have suffered tissue loss and those that have not. Wounds that have not lost tissue are those caused by sharp lacerations, e.g. surgical incisions. Avulsion injuries, crush injuries, bite wounds and burns will lead to deep as well as surface tissue destruction. The severity of the wound affects factors such as the duration of healing and the probability of complications.

The most important question to ask about a wound is whether closure is possible without complications (see Chapter 4). To answer this it is essential to consider the degree of contamination that will indicate the likelihood of wound infection developing (Figure 5.1), remembering that contamination does not imply infection. The presence of blood, breakdown products of haemoglobin, dirt and devitalized tissue will provide an ideal environment for bacterial multiplication. This not only provides a source for bacterial nutrition but also inhibits the effective functioning of neutrophils. It is important to consider the time from the traumatic incident to presentation. The expression 'golden period' is often quoted, the time interval which, historically, has been described as being a safe period in which to close a wound primarily. Such an all-encompassing time interval makes no allowance for local blood supply to the wound, the degree of contamination or the extent of tissue injuries. Each wound must be evaluated individually. If there is any doubt, it is best to assume that the wound is contaminated, to manage it as an open wound and to consider surgical closure at a later stage.

Open wound management allows for continued wound drainage, regular wound inspection, lavage and debridement as required. Finally a decision can be made as to the preferred closure technique once all contamination and devitalized tissue have been removed. This is summarized in Figure 5.2.

WOUND LAVAGE

Wound lavage is an essential part of wound management as it significantly reduces bacterial numbers as well as removing free foreign material. The pressure required for adequate lavage is between 4 and 15

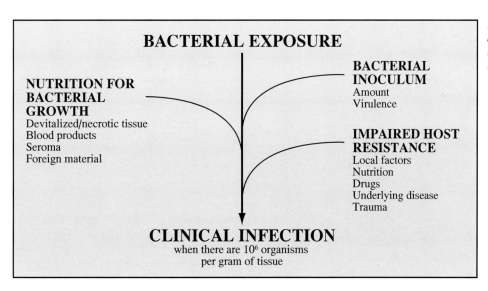

BACTERIAL EXPOSURE

NUTRITION FOR BACTERIAL GROWTH
Devitalized/necrotic tissue
Blood products
Seroma
Foreign material

BACTERIAL INOCULUM
Amount
Virulence

IMPAIRED HOST RESISTANCE
Local factors
Nutrition
Drugs
Underlying disease
Trauma

CLINICAL INFECTION
when there are 10^6 organisms
per gram of tissue

Figure 5.1: Factors that determine whether bacterial exposure results in infection.

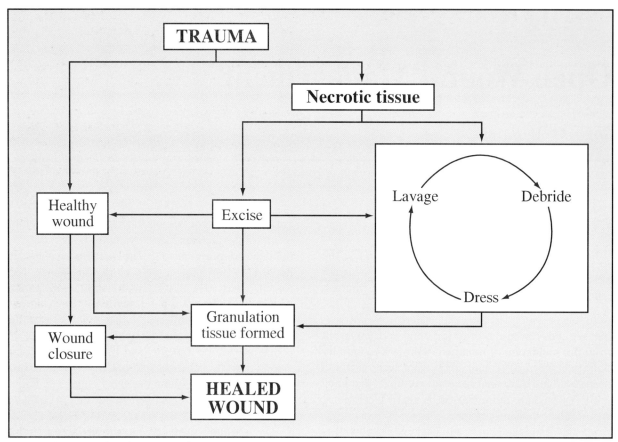

Figure 5.2: Steps to be taken in wound management.

pounds per square inch (psi). A pressure of 8 psi can be achieved using a 20–30 ml syringe, adapted for rapid refilling by attachment to the distal end of an intravenous giving set via a three-way tap (Figure 5.3). High pressure lavage should not be used, e.g. water-pik type instruments (at the mid or high setting these will produce 40–50 psi), as this will drive debris and bacteria further into the tissues. Ideally a sterile isotonic solution should be used, e.g. Hartmann's (lactated Ringer's) solution.

There is some debate as to whether or not to add antiseptic solutions to the lavage solution. As it is the physical flushing of the wound that is important, it is likely that their addition is not essential. Tap water has been used as a readily available alternative to isotonic solutions and can be delivered via a shower head attachment. However, recent work has shown that tap water is not ideal as it is cytotoxic to fibroblasts, due to its alkaline pH, hypotonicity, and the presence of various trace elements. Perhaps surprisingly, the same report indicated that normal saline is also cytotoxic, due to its lack of a buffering system and its acid pH. Thus Hartmann's solution would seem to be the ideal lavage solution as it has no cytotoxic effects. If an antiseptic is felt to be necessary then it should be used at very low concentrations so as not to interfere with the healing process. Chlorhexidine should be used at a concentration of 0.05% (a 1 in 40 dilution)

and povidone–iodine at 1%. Chlorhexidine appears to be superior to povidone–iodine in minimizing wound infection, and its ability to bind to surface proteins provides it with prolonged residual activity. Povidone–iodine has very limited residual activity in the presence of organic matter, and its value must therefore be questioned in managing contaminated wounds. Similarly the addition of topical antibiotics has no advantage over systemic antibiotics as the latter will readily and rapidly achieve high local tissue concentrations.

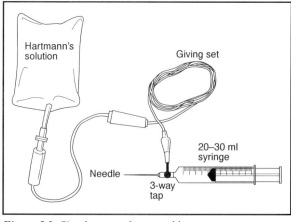

Figure 5.3: Simple set-up for wound lavage.

TOPICAL WOUND MANAGEMENT

Antibiotics

There is little positive value in the use of topical antibiotics in open wound management especially if there is ongoing infection. Antibiotics are a poor substitute for aggressive wound lavage and debridement.

Antiseptics

The antiseptics chlorhexidine and povidone–iodine have been discussed earlier under wound lavage.

Hydrogels/hydroactive dressings

Hydrogels can be considered as topical wound agents and are probably the most exciting development in open wound management over the past decade. They are available as commercial wound dressings. The concept of hydroactive dressings will be considered in detail in the section on dressings (see below).

Honey

Honey was reported as an effective topical wound agent by the Egyptians in *c.* 1600 BC (this was descibed in the so-called Edwin Smith papyrus; *c.* AD 1700). It has two positive effects: it is bacteriostatic and it helps with wound cleansing. The former is a function of the low pH (~ 3.7) which is achieved at the wound surface; this has been shown to kill and inhibit streptococci and coagulase-positive staphylococci. Honey has been shown to take 3–6 days to render a wound sterile in human clinical studies. The cleansing effect of honey is due to its high osmotic pressure which draws fluid from the tissues. It is likely that honey has a role to play in wound management, though there are few reports of its use in veterinary wounds. It can be considered as an alternative to hydrogels where cost is an issue.

Enzymatic debriding agents

Enzymatic debridement is relatively selective in removing necrotic tissue and its loosening effect on necrotic debris may avoid the need for surgical debridement. The agents used act on collagen, protein, fibrin, elastin and/or nucleoproteins. The precise method of action depends on the product being used. Tunnelling wounds and sinuses would seem particularly suitable for these products as they remove debris which may be difficult to visualize or reach surgically. In the UK there are no licensed veterinary topical enzymatic agents, though a number of human preparations are available on prescription, e.g. streptokinase/streptodornase. In the USA a commonly used enzymatic debriding agent is sutilains ointment derived from *Bacillus subtilis*. Their role has always been limited in veterinary wound management and in human wound management their use has been supplanted by the hydrogels.

Sodium hypochlorite (Dakin's solution)

Solutions of sodium hypochlorite normally have a pH of 11 and are highly irritant but when suitably buffered (as Dakin's solution) can be used as a lavage and cleansing agent. During World War I it was used extensively and helped in reducing wound sepsis and dissolution of necrotic debris. When used it is at a strength of 0.125–0.25%, and there is concern that even at such dilutions significant cytotoxicity occurs. The use of such a potentially irritating solution has declined dramatically with the advent of antibiotics and especially the hydrogels.

Organic acids

Products containing benzoic acid, malic acid, salicylic acid and propylene glycol are used extensively as wound cleansing and debriding agents. The mode of action is by achieving separation following differential swelling of necrotic and healthy tissue, this being achieved by the low pH of the solution and the reaction of the organic acids in separating collagen chains. Their efficacy has been questioned and, with hydrogels being able to achieve gentler autolysis, their role in the future will be limited.

Larval therapy

In human wound management larval therapy (with maggots) is becoming increasingly popular as a means of gently debriding wounds. The concept has been around for several hundred years and the practice only waned during the 1940s with the advent of antibiotics. The most popular larvae are those of *Lucilia sericata*, the greenbottle fly. The greenbottle eggs are collected and cleaned aseptically to allow the larvae to hatch in a sterile environment; they are then stored in a cool environment until they are required.

Skin surrounding the wound is protected by strips of a hydrocolloid sheet approximately 2 cm wide. About 10 larvae per cm^2 of wound area are introduced into the wound and held in place by a piece of sterile net trimmed to overlap the edges of the wound by about 1 cm. The net is attached to the hydrocolloid dressing with adhesive tape, ensuring the edge is completely sealed to prevent the maggots escaping.

The hydrocolloid frame provides anchoring for the net, and protects the skin around the wound from the action of the proteolytic enzymes produced by the larvae. It also stops the larvae from migrating on to intact skin. Moistened gauze swabs or a hydrocolloid dressing are placed on the outside of the net to prevent the larvae from drying out.

The 'dressing' is left in place for 48–72 hours, after which time the larvae are washed off the wound and the wound reassessed. Such treatment is remarkably well tolerated by people and its use could be considered for veterinary wounds where there are particularly large amounts of necrotic tissue present. The larvae have powerful enzymatic systems, which have yet to be fully characterized.

Miscellaneous agents

Hydrogen peroxide, wound powders and intra-mammary antibiotic preparations have no positive value in wound management and their use should be discouraged. Hydrogen peroxide damages cells, especially the capillary bed, and significantly delays healing. Wound powders also significantly delay healing as they are essentially foreign particles which must be cleared by inflammatory cells, and they predispose to foreign body granuloma formation.

SURGICAL DEBRIDEMENT

Following copious lavage of the wound, further gross necrotic material and debris should be removed by carrying out surgical debridement. This can be defined as the removal of dirt, foreign objects, damaged tissue and cellular debris from a wound, so as to minimize infection and promote healing.

Wound debridement should be considered a surgical procedure and strict aseptic techniques employed. In many instances general anaesthesia should be used to allow for proper preparation of the patient and a thorough evaluation of the wound.

1. A wide area is clipped around the wound with a No. 40 clipper blade
2. The wound is packed with a water-soluble jelly or saline-soaked swabs to prevent clipped hair from contaminating the wound
3. The gel is rinsed or wiped out with sterile swabs after clipping
4. The clipped area should be prepared with a suitable antiseptic.

No alcohol or detergent-based antiseptic solutions should be used as they may delay the healing process. Detergents should never be used in conjunction with povidone–iodine as they may combine to form surfactants which damage tissue and enhance infection.

En bloc debridement is used to describe the complete wide local excision of a contaminated wound followed by primary closure of the resultant clean deficit. This is a technique rarely used in veterinary patients. It can be used on the trunk or proximal limbs but there is rarely enough tissue in distal limbs to allow this to be carried out. The major advantage of this technique is that it allows for primary wound closure and therefore will reduce time and cost in management of an open wound (Figure 5.4).

The surgical procedure most commonly carried out is *layered* debridement. This begins by excising devitalized tissue, and removing any debris at the surface, and progresses to the deeper tissues (Figure 5.5). A scalpel is preferred to scissors as it produces a sharper incision and tissue is cut back until it bleeds. Haemorrhage is an indication of healthy tissue. If there is doubt

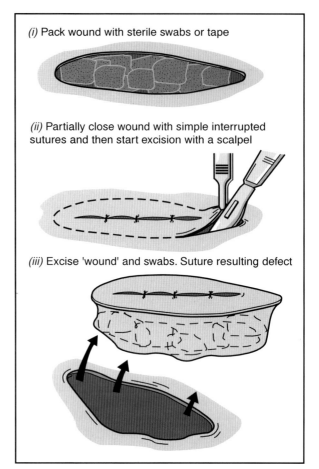

(i) Pack wound with sterile swabs or tape

(ii) Partially close wound with simple interrupted sutures and then start excision with a scalpel

(iii) Excise 'wound' and swabs. Suture resulting defect

Figure 5.4: En bloc *wound debridement.*

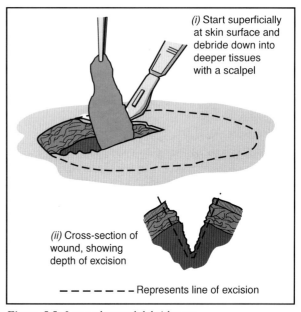

(i) Start superficially at skin surface and debride down into deeper tissues with a scalpel

(ii) Cross-section of wound, showing depth of excision

– – – – – – Represents line of excision

Figure 5.5: *Layered wound debridement.*

over an area of tissue, it should be excised. In distal extremities there is some merit in managing the wound with dressing (see below) for 2–3 days until a clear demarcation exists between healthy and necrotic tissue. Keeping as much tissue as possible is of vital importance for large deficits where as much skin and other tissues as possible should be preserved in order to allow closure.

SYSTEMIC MEDICATION

At the time of presentation a wound is likely to be contaminated and the use of systemic antibiotics should be considered. Ideally antibiotics should be used to prevent bacterial multiplication but with traumatic wounds the level of contamination may already be significant and therefore antibiotics are relied on to help reduce the number of bacteria. If they are to be used prophylactically then they must be administered within 3 hours of the trauma. It must always be remembered that antimicrobial prophylaxis is not a substitute for effective lavage, debridement and dressings. The choice of antibiotic should ideally be based on the results of bacterial culture and sensitivity; as these will not be known at the time of presentation a suitable broad spectrum antibiotic can be used which is effective against the most likely contaminants in the wound, which will be either coagulase-positive staphylococci or *Escherichia coli*. A rough indication of the contaminants can be obtained by performing a Gram stain on a direct smear from the wound. The choice of antibiotic must also take into account the potential risk of infection and its consequence and the cost of the antibiotic. The preferred antibiotics to use are clavulanic acid-potentiated amoxycillin, second-generation cephalosporins or fluoroquinolones. The antibiotic can be changed if the results of culture and sensitivity dictate this. It is also worthwhile considering the basic actions of antibiotics when making a choice, for example:

- Pseudomonads are resistant to β-lactam antimicrobials as well as first- and second-generation cephalosporins
- Potentiated sulphonamides have very poor activity against abscesses and areas of grossly necrotic tissue
- Anaerobes are generally resistant to fluoroquinolones and aminoglycosides.

It is best to have a few well chosen antibiotics and to use them routinely, rather than use a wide range of drugs. The justification for continued anti-biosis beyond the first 24 hours is questionable, as persistent use may predispose to nosocomial super-infection with organisms such as pseudomanads and *Klebsiella* spp.

BANDAGING PRINCIPLES FOR WOUND MANAGEMENT

The role of bandaging in open wound management is to provide an environment in which optimal wound contraction and epithelialization can occur. The functions of a bandage and dressing are to:

- Exert pressure for dead space obliteration and reduction of oedema and haemorrhage
- Pack a wound
- Debride a wound and absorb exudate
- Protect the wound from environmental bacteria
- Immobilize the wound and support adjacent osseous structures
- Provide comfort
- Act as a vehicle for antibiotics and antiseptics.

Generally bandages have three basic component layers (Figure 5.6):

- Primary (Contact) layer
- Secondary (Intermediate) layer
- Tertiary (Outer) layer.

Primary (contact) layer

The contact layer is critical in that when correctly chosen it allows for optimal healing. Optimal healing has been shown to occur under the following conditions:

- Moist (not too wet and macerated)
- No infection/necrosis
- No toxins/particles/loose fibres
- Optimum temperature (35–37°C)
- Undisturbed
- Minimal infection
- pH is maintained around 6 which inhibits bacterial multiplication.

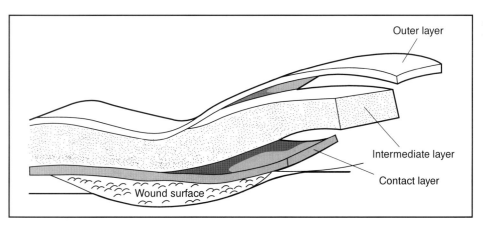

Figure 5.6: The layers of a bandage.

Outer layer

Intermediate layer

Contact layer

Wound surface

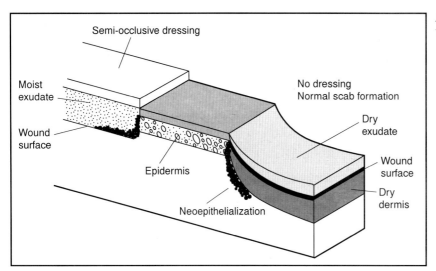

Figure 5.7: Moist versus dry wound healing.

Modern semi-occlusive dressings will allow many of these criteria to be achieved. Since the early 1960s it has been accepted that wounds which are kept moist (Figure 5.7) will heal more rapidly by up to 40% compared to wounds allowed to dry out.

The primary layer must be sterile and remain in close contact with the surface of the wound while the patient is either resting or moving. If any space is present between the dressing and the wound, drainage is likely to be impaired and tissue maceration may occur. It is essential that this layer therefore conforms to the body contours. In wounds which are exudative or draining it is essential that the contact layer allows fluid to pass through to the secondary or absorbent layer of the dressing. Dressings applied to non-exudative wounds should prevent exogenous contamination. Meshed materials should be fine enough to prevent penetration by fibrinous tissue. The contact layer should minimize pain, prevent unnecessary loss of body fluid, and be non-toxic and non-irritating to tissues.

Adherent contact layer

Adherence to the wound is only indicated early on in wound healing (debridement stage). At this stage a decision must be made whether to apply dry or wet dressings, depending on the amount of exudate/transudate coming from the wound. Such dressings are useful in further debriding a wound once gross debris and necrotic tissues have been removed surgically.

Adherence occurs by one of two mechanisms:

- Proteinaceous exudate penetrates the dressing, which then dries by absorption into the secondary layer

  OR

- There is penetration of the dressing mesh by granulation tissue; an indication that the dressing has been left in place for too long.

Dry-to-dry dressings: These are reserved for wounds which still have considerable amounts of foreign debris or loose necrotic tissue which is not amenable to further surgical debridement. Alternatively they may be applied to wounds that possess large volumes of low-viscosity exudate which does not tend to aggregate. Dry sterile gauze swabs have a good absorptive capacity, allowing debris and necrotic material to adhere to them. The bandage should be left in place until both the contact and intermediate layers have absorbed exudate and the primary dressing has dried. Removal of the contact layer results in debridement of the wound. Dry-to-dry dressings are by their nature extremely painful to remove from wounds since they tend to remove viable as well as necrotic tissue. In some instances it may be preferable either to infiltrate the dressing with a local anaesthetic during removal or to anaesthetize the patient. Because of the length of time required to dry the primary layer, there is increased risk with dry-to-dry dressings of granulation tissue infiltrating between the mesh of the gauze. With the advent of hydrogel dressing materials dry-to-dry dressings are now rarely indicated.

Wet-to-dry dressings: Wet-to-dry dressings have historically been the mainstay of early wound management where there is viscous exudate plus necrotic tissue and debris. They also serve to preserve the moist environment which is preferred for wound healing. The sterile gauze is preferably soaked in sterile Hartmann's solution, though both sterile isotonic saline and water have been advocated in the past. The majority of the fluid is then squeezed out and the dressing applied to the wound; this is followed by an absorbent secondary layer and a tertiary layer, which will allow some evaporation. The water in the gauze dilutes the exudate, allowing its absorption; as the dressing dries out, debris and necrotic material will adhere to it (Figure 5.8). Such dressings need to be changed at least every 24 hours and more often if there are copious amounts of exudate present. There may be some pain and discomfort on removal. If too wet, such

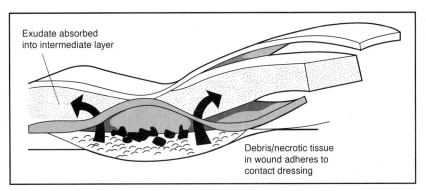

Exudate absorbed
into intermediate layer

Debris/necrotic tissue
in wound adheres to
contact dressing

Figure 5.8: Wet-to-dry dressing.

a dressing may allow tissue maceration or bacterial strikethrough as bacteria flourish in the wet local environment. Because of this risk some authors advocate the use of antiseptics in the wetting solution, such as 0.05% chlorhexidine solution.

Recently hydrogels (see below) have been advocated as a suitable alternative 'wetting' agent. Their advantage is an increased absorptive capacity, they act as a desloughing agent and allow for a much gentler debridement when the dressing is removed. These products also reduce the number of dressing changes required. Hydrogels can also be applied under absorptive non-adherent dressings and debride the wound equally well. The amorphous hydrogels can be left in place for 48 hours with most wounds, which reduces the number of dressing changes required. The appearance of the gels at the time of dressing change often resembles pus, and clients should be warned of this if they are present during dressing changes. This is the normal appearance of hydrogels following fluid absorption.

Non-adherent contact layer

Once granulation tissue is forming, and prior to epithelialization, the contact dressing should not be allowed to adhere to the wound, but should be able to absorb exudate. The use of hydrogels in the amorphous form or as sheets has changed our approach once granulation is present as there is no real need to change the type of dressing. However if a classical wet-to-dry or dry-to-dry dressing has been used, it is essential to change to a non-adherent contact layer.

Early non-adherent dressings

Classically such a dressing is wide meshed gauze impregnated with petroleum jelly. Such dressing should *not* be used if there is evidence of peripheral epithelialization as the jelly reduces oxygen tension in the wound and therefore delays epithelialization. This is a very small window of opportunity and given the wide range of excellent non-adherent semi-occlusive dressing now available for open wound management, there are few if any indications for the use of these older products.

Late non-adherent dressings

Absorbent semi-occlusive non-adhering dressings maintain a moist wound without reducing oxygen

tension and can therefore be used in the presence of epithelialization. Such dressings have an outer semi-permeable polyethylene film with some form of absorbent layer and they allow absorption of wound exudate whilst maintaining adequate oxygen levels at the wound surface to allow re-epithelialization. These dressings are to a greater or lesser degree non-adherent. Figure 5.9 shows some of the products available.

Type of dressing	Trade name	Manufacturer
Perforated film absorbent dressings	Melolin Release Skintact Cutilin	Smith & Nephew Johnson & Johnson Robinson Healthcare TSK Animal Health
Foam dressings	Lyofoam Cutinova Foam Tielle Allevyn	Ultra Laboratories Ltd TSK Animal Health Johnson & Johnson Smith & Nephew
Hydrogels	Intrasite Granugel Nu-Gel AquaFoam Cutinova Cavity Cutinova Hydro Biodres	Smith & Nephew ConvaTec Johnson & Johnson TSK Animal Health TSK Animal Health TSK Animal Health DVM Pharmaceuticals
Hydrocolloid dressings	Tegasorb Granuflex Comfeel	3M ConvaTec Coloplast Ltd
Alginate dressings	Kaltogel Kaltostat AlgiSite Algosteril Sorbsan Tegagel	ConvaTec ConvaTec Smith & Nephew TSK Animal Health Animalcare Ltd 3M
Semi-permeable adhesive film	Cutifilm Opsite Tegaderm Bioclusive	BDF Medical Ltd Smith & Nephew 3M Johnson & Johnson

Figure 5.9: A guide to commercially available wound dressing products. This list is not designed to be comprehensive or exhaustive, but is an indication of what is available.

Perforated film dressings: Regrettably, apart from semipermeable films and hydroactive dressing materials the majority of contact dressings show some tendency to adhere to the surface of the wound. The films that are applied to the dressing surface to reduce adherence are essentially sheets of plastic with microscopic pores. The size and number of these pores is critical for the success of these dressings. Below a critical size, wound exudate will stay on the wound surface and will predispose to local inflammation under the dressing itself. It is also common with such perforated film dressings to find secondary damage at the site of the pores due to local dehydration secondary to moisture evaporation. Such problems have now been largely overcome by the development of foam-based dressings.

Foam dressings: These are a recent development in wound mangement, produced in order to overcome the limitations of the earlier perforated film dressings. One commercial multi-layered product has a perforated non-adherent polyurethane film, a polyurethane foam, hydrophilic core and an outer polyurethane film; this has excellent absorptive capacity and maintains a warm (35°C) moist well oxygenated environment. The major advantage of this product is the large absorptive capacity of the foam (1400 g/m²/24h) even when compressed. The backing layer also allows controlled evaporation and acts as a very effective bacterial barrier. The capacity of the foam and the backing layer are such that it prevents dehydration at the wound surface and therefore minimizes any risk of adherence or localized dehydration at the pore site of the surface polyurethane film.

Hydroactive dressings: Hydroactive dressings have become one of the major ways of dealing with open wounds in that they aid moist wound healing, allowing autolysis and debridement. These dressings fall into three basic categories, namely amorphous hydrogels, sheet hydrogels and hydrocolloids. Alginates by their activity can also be considered as hydrocolloids.

Essentially hydrogels consist of insoluble polymers, which have the ability to absorb and retain large volumes of water following interaction with aqueous solutions or wound exudate. The amorphous hydrogels have shown themselves to be particularly effective in the management of wounds with necrotic tissue and debris present (Figure 5.10) The gel rehydrates dead tissue and allows normal autolytic processes to debride the wound. Amorphous hydrogels will not only swell but tend to flow to the shape of the wound as they reduce in viscosity. Some earlier workers added antibiotics such as metronidazole to the product but it is now felt that this is largely unnecessary, as the hydrogel itself has a significant antibacterial activity. Amorphous hydrogels are particularly suited to wounds with large defects and cavities. They do need to be applied with a suitable secondary dressing to keep them in place.

Sheet hydrogels have a fixed three-dimensional structure, this does not change its physical form but will swell due to fluid absorption.

Hydrocolloids: Hydrocolloids comprise a self-adhesive gel of carboxymethylcellulose and usually gelatin, and are held in place by a thin polyurethane or foam sheet. Initially the hydrocolloids are totally impervious to water and are therefore extremely valuable in rehydrating a wound to precipitate autolysis and debridement. As the gel forms the product becomes more water permeable and allows fluid to escape from the dressing; this allows the hydrocolloids to cope with moderate amounts of wound exudate though they cannot manage large volumes.

Hydrocolloid dressings are ideal products where there is superficial injury with minimal exudate or they can be used to secure a hydrogel or alginate in place. Thin hydrocolloids are associated with very low infection rates at the wound site; due to low local pH and the fact that the dressing is impervious to bacteria, it would appear to be particularly effective in reducing local infection with *Pseudomonas aeruginosa*. There is relatively rapid wound healing, which may be due to a high concentration of wound cytokines trapped by the dressing at the surface. There is minimal pain associated with its use or removal. Hydrocolloids are effective in enhancing autolytic wound debridement due to maintenance of a moist wound surface as with all hydroactive dressings and need only be changed twice a week.

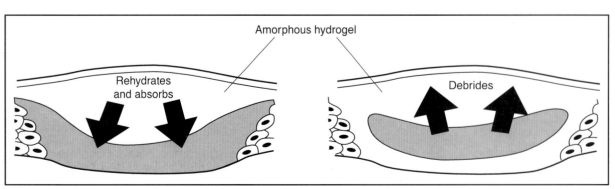

Figure 5.10: *Amorphous hydrogel rehydrates, debrides via autolysis and absorbs necrotic tissue.*

Sheet hydrocolloids adhere to normal skin surface while the area over the wound interacts to form a non-adherent gel. This type of dressing is designed to be applied to moderately exudative wounds through to granulating wounds. The dressing should be left in place for 2–3 days; such a product not only encourages desloughing and debriding but will predispose to rapid epithelialization and reduced wound contraction.

A hydroactive dressing is, in this author's opinion, one of the most valuable materials that can be applied to a wound, either in sheet or amorphous form. The only real disadvantage, apart from cost, is that hydroactive dressings should not be used directly on wounds which are highly exudative though the sheet hydrocolloids can be used as secondary dressings over a primary dressing such as an alginate.

Alginates: Alginate dressings are possibly the most underused and undervalued of all the primary wound dressings available. They are generally woven products, of both calcium and sodium alginate, derived from brown seaweeds (e.g. giant kelp). Calcium alginate is relatively insoluble but will form a gel in the presence of sodium ions. These may be provided by the wound exudate or are included in the dressing itself; the advantage of the mixed salts is that they tend to form a gel more rapidly. The gel formed is extremely hydrophilic, which aids moist wound healing and promotes autolysis. The absorptive capacity of alginate swabs is some three times that of an equivalent-sized gauze swab. They also appear to allow rapid healing with minimal wound discomfort, when the wound is exudative. There is some evidence that calcium alginate may promote formation of fibroblasts and thus actively aid in the healing process. There is no pain associated with their removal due to the gel formation. In cases where there is minimal exudation, a non-adherent dressing should be placed over the dressing. In general, alginate dressings need only be changed every 2–3 days. Alginates have both haemostatic and absorptive properties. The haemostatic activity is believed to be due to exchange of calcium and sodium ions in the blood, allowing activation of platelets and coagulation. An alginate should not be placed in deep wounds or within body cavities as it can set up a severe foreign body reaction, they are not designed as absorbable haemostatic agents for intraoperative use.

Semipermeable film dressings: Granulating wounds with little or no exudate can be dressed with an adhesive polyurethane film which acts as an excellent semi-occlusive dressing, maintaining moisture at the surface and thereby encouraging epithelialization. The main problem with dogs and cats is non-adherence to the normal skin.

Secondary (intermediate) layer

It is essential that all layers of a bandage are correctly and meticulously applied in order to avoid the common complications that can arise from inadequate, unskilled or incorrect application. The role of the secondary layer in wound management, in addition to providing support and comfort, is absorption. It acts as a 'trap' for exudative fluids from the wound, evaporation from this layer helps prevent bacterial strikethrough. To aid its absorptive role this layer needs to have good capillarity and should be thick enough (single or preferably multi-layered) to collect the fluid and pad the wound. The intermediate layer must be in close contact with the primary dressing but it should not be applied so tightly as to limit exudate absorption (Figure 5.11). Suitable materials are hospital-quality absorbent cotton wool, or synthetic materials.

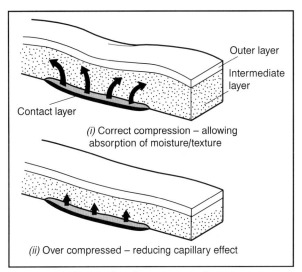

Figure 5.11: Intermediate layer compression.

Tertiary (outer) layer

The outer layer serves to hold all the other layers of the bandage in place. In a multi-layered bandage (e.g. modified Robert Jones), intermediate layers of conforming gauze and absorbent material may be used prior to applying an outer covering such as an adhesive wrap or preferably a self-adhering dressing. It is important that the outer layer allows evaporation of fluid but minimizes external fluid absorption. Plastic bags which may be placed over the distal dressing should only be left *in situ* for a minimal period to prevent excessive fluid retention with the increased risk of bacterial strikethrough and tissue maceration.

Tie-over (bolus) dressings

Tie-over (bolus) dressings are a useful method of securing contact layers to parts of the body, where conventional bandaging techniques are of limited value, e.g. over the greater trochanter. The most common

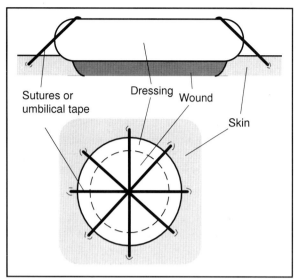

Sutures or umbilical tape   Dressing Wound

Skin

Figure 5.12: Tie-over bolus dressing.

method of securing such a dressing is to use loops of 3m (2/0) monofilament nylon sutures that are placed some 2 cm from the wound edge. Umbilical (nylon) tape is passed through these loops to secure the dressing (Figure 5.12).

Non-adherent dressing is applied to the wound, and cotton wool is then placed in the centre of the dressing. The edges of the dressing are then folded over and secured either with sutures or umbilical tape. Recently the author has used an amorphous hydrogel covered by a non-adherent foam dressing which was held in place by umbilical tape to good effect.

Pressure relief bandages

Pressure relief dressings are indicated for decubital ulcer type lesions or superficial ulceration secondary to bandages or casts. Generally doughnut-shaped and pipe insulation bandages are employed to protect the area concerned. Care should be taken when using doughnut-shaped bandages, as they can in some instances be counterproductive as they produce a 'halo' compression of the skin around a bony prominence. This compression can occasionally be severe enough to compromise the circulation and therefore delay healing. Soft foam pad (pipe insulation) can be used parallel to the lesion so as not to encircle the wound and therefore not compromise the circulation.

FURTHER READING

Pavletic M (1990) Plastic and Reconstructive Surgery. *Veterinary Clinics of North America: Small Animal Practice* **20**

Pavletic M (1993) *Atlas of Small Animal Reconstructive Surgery.* Lippincott, Philadelphia

Swaim SF and Henderson RA (1997) *Small Animal Wound Management, 2nd edn.* Williams and Wilkins, Baltimore

Thomas S (1990) *Wound Management and Dressings.* The Pharmaceutical Press, London

Further information on wound dressings can be obtained from the Surgical Materials Testing Laboratory, Bridgend General Hospital, Mid-Glamorgan website at http://www.smtl.co.uk

CHAPTER SIX

Surgical Drains

Stephen J. Baines

INTRODUCTION

This chapter will review the types of drains available, the indications for their use in wound management and reconstruction, and potential complications. Some controversy still exists over the effectiveness, therapeutic indications, applications and maintenance requirements of drains. This is due, in part, to the fact that their value depends on both the method of application and case selection.

GENERAL INDICATIONS

A drain is a temporary surgical implant which provides and maintains a channel of exit for the purpose of removing fluids (blood, serum, exudate), foreign material and air from a wound or body cavity. The correct application of drains will reduce the wound infection rate and shorten the healing time. However, the misapplication of drains increases morbidity and mortality.

Surgical drains have two main indications:

- To eliminate the potential for dead space
- To remove fluid accumulation from a wound.

Elimination of dead space
Dead space is an abnormal space within a wound, containing fluid or gas. Wounds involving extensive subcutaneous dissection, created by removal of a large mass or reconstructed with skin grafts or flaps will contain an appreciable amount of dead space. Elimination of dead space promotes early union of divided tissues. Dead space may be eliminated by:

- Surgical means: e.g. tacking sutures
- Pressure bandages
- Surgical drains.

Surgical drains can and should be used in conjunction with the other two methods. If dead space can be eliminated using the first two methods, then drains should not be used. However, these methods have their own inherent disadvantages.

Surgical reduction of dead space may not be sufficient, may risk damage to the underlying structures by sutures, and may increase the wound infection rate because of implanted foreign material and potential damage to the blood supply of the tissue. Surgical closure of dead space alone is not advocated for routine use in contaminated wounds. In addition, if a seroma does form, the presence of buried tacking sutures results in the formation of many, smaller pockets, which do not communicate with each other. This makes it difficult to establish drainage.

Pressure bandages may only supply pressure for a few hours, may apply excessive pressure resulting in compromised blood supply, or may be inappropriate for certain sites (e.g. head and neck).

Removal of fluid accumulation from a wound
Fluid accumulation within a wound reduces host resistance to infection and reduces healing by the following mechanisms:

- The opsonic activity of antibodies is progressively lost in fluid
- Fluid interferes with the access of phagocytes to bacteria
- Fluid provides a substrate for bacterial growth
- Wound fluid may compromise the blood supply to the surrounding tissue
- Fluid accumulation may interfere with graft acceptance.

The use of surgical drains is indicated where:

- Fluid accumulation will recur after simple evacuations, e.g. large seromas
- Fluid cannot be readily removed, e.g. abscesses
- Wounds cannot be completely debrided, and contain foreign material or necrotic debris
- Fluid will remain or be produced after surgery, e.g. salivary mucocoele, skin flap
- Massive contamination is inevitable, e.g. perianal wounds.

Wound factors	Is there a need for drainage? What type of discharge is present or expected (viscosity, volume)? What type of wound is present? Where is the wound located?
Patient factors	Will the patient tolerate the presence of a drain?
Hospital environment	What drains are available? What standard of postoperative care will be available?
Drainage system	Which type of drain will be most effective? Is an active or passive drain indicated?
Cost	Use the most cost-effective for the type of wound

Figure 6.1: Factors affecting the choice of surgical drain.

Another frequently quoted, but wholly unsubstantiated, role for drains is their prophylactic placement as a means of detecting fluid accumulation within a wound. The prophylactic use of drains is not a substitute for good surgical technique and careful patient evaluation. The use of drains is not without the risk of complications and other more satisfactory and less invasive methods of detecting fluid accumulations exist. Hence surgical drains should not be used in this manner.

CHOICE OF SURGICAL DRAIN

General guidelines rather than absolute rules exist; it is important to evaluate each patient individually. The factors in Figure 6.1 need to be considered to ensure that the drainage system is a success.

TYPE AND TECHNIQUE OF DRAINAGE

In addition to the use of surgical implants it is important to realize that wound drainage may also be achieved by the following means:

- Open wound drainage, i.e. the wound is not closed
- Fenestration of part of the skin surface, e.g. meshed skin grafts
- Use of a physiological implant, e.g. placing of omentum.

Surgical drainage systems may be classified by the following characteristics:

- Mechanism of action: passive or active
- Type of implant: surface-acting or tube drain
- Suction system: commercially available or 'home-made'

Mechanism of action

Passive drainage

Passive drains provide a path of least resistance to the exterior and function chiefly by overflow of fluid from the wound. They are assisted by gravity and are influenced by pressure differentials within the wound, which may be induced by normal tissue movement or by a pressure bandage. Fluid normally passes over the surface of the drain and therefore a drain's efficacy is largely dictated by its surface area. Passive drains placed non-dependently lose their efficacy. Passive drains placed in certain locations (e.g. the axillary and inguinal regions) may allow air to be sucked into the wound as the tissues move, resulting in emphysema.

The most widely used passive drains are the Penrose drain (Figure 6.2) and the corrugated drain (Figure 6.3).

Active drainage

An active drain uses an external source of suction to remove fluid from the wound. Suction increases the efficiency of dependently placed drains and can remove fluid against the influence of gravity. Suction drains are of use if dependent drainage is difficult to obtain or where the patient's posture frequently alters the point of dependency. They are also of more use if large volumes of fluid are expected.

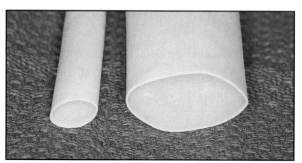

Figure 6.2: Penrose drain.

Copyright © R.A.S. White.

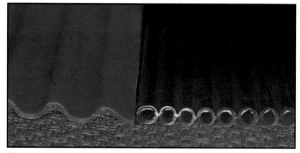

Figure 6.3: Corrugated drain (left) and Yeates drain (right).

Copyright © R.A.S. White.

Closed suction: This uses negative pressure applied to a single-lumen drain with no air vent. This allows the wound and dressing to be kept dry, prevents bacteria ascending via the drain and markedly reduces the infection rate. The incidence of postoperative haematoma and seroma is also reduced compared with passive drains. Closed suction drains help keep skin flaps in apposition to the wound bed and result in early revascularization and enhanced healing (Pope and Swaim, 1986).

Vented suction: This uses a continuous source of suction and a multi-lumen drain (sump drain) and is the most efficient way of removing large volumes of fluid. High-volume suction (20 l/min) is more likely to result in wound contamination than low-volume suction (4 l/min). In addition, a large volume of air moving through the wound may be traumatic to the tissues. This volume of suction requires that the drain is attached to a wall-mounted or mobile suction generator. For these reasons, vented suction has little use in the management of wounds in small animals (Swaim and Lee, 1990).

Correctly applied suction will create an 'atmospheric bandage' sufficient to obliterate the dead space without damaging tissues. Suction may be applied continuously or intermittently (at least every 6 hours). Continuous suction is more effective, and more useful where high volumes of fluid are anticipated. The continuous, uninterrupted flow reduces the likelihood of drain occlusion and results in a shorter period of drainage. Intermittent suction allows the system to be secured between suction episodes, reducing the risk of inadvertent disconnection. Ideally, the suction device should incorporate a one-way valve to prevent reflux of fluid from the reservoir into the wound.

The suction device may be a portable reservoir, which is taped, sutured or attached to the patient with a bandage, or a wall-mounted or mobile suction generator. The former are more convenient and more widely used in wound management, and may consist of a commercially available reservoir or may be 'home-made'.

Commercial reservoirs consist of either a rigid evacuated container or a flexible, compressible receptacle (Figure 6.4). Commercially available units are convenient to use, are less likely to become detached and operate at lower pressures (80 mmHg) than home-made devices, thus reducing the risk of tissue trauma and occlusion or collapse of the tube.

Home-made devices may be constructed using a 10 ml evacuated glass tube (Figure 6.5) or a large (30 or 60 ml) syringe (Lee *et al.*, 1986) (Figure 6.6).

The evacuated glass tube is combined with a butterfly scalp needle. The syringe adapter is detached, the extension tubing is fenestrated and implanted into the

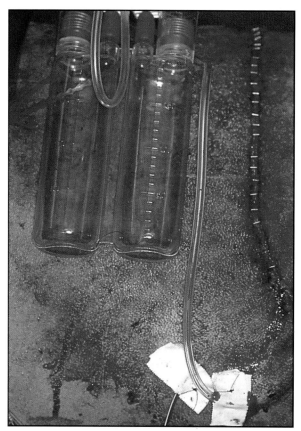

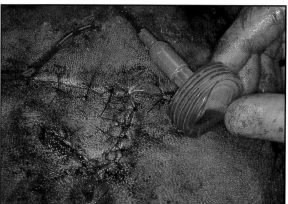

Figure 6.4: *Two types of commercial suction device.*

wound (Figure 6.5a). On wound closure the needle is introduced into the evacuated tube to provide suction (Figure 6.5b).

If a syringe is used, it is attached to the tube drain and the plunger retracted until the desired pressure is achieved. A pin or 18-gauge needle is then inserted through the plunger, above the syringe barrel, so retaining it in place (Figure 6.6). The tip of the needle or pin must be covered or blunted so that it will not traumatize the patient.

Small blood tubes are effective and less cumbersome to handle and incorporate into a bandage than a syringe. However, they are more fragile and may need to be changed several times a day in highly productive wounds.

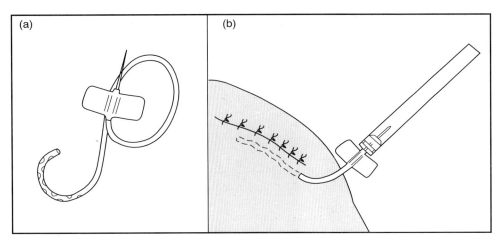

Figure 6.5: 'Home-made' suction device using an evacuated glass tube and butterfly needle. (a) A 19-gauge butterfly needle with multiple fenestrations; the Luer–Lock attachment has been removed from the extension tubing. (b) Placement of drain and connection of suction device.

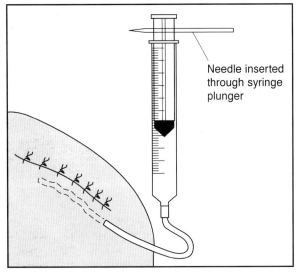

Needle inserted through syringe plunger

Figure 6.6: 'Home-made' suction device using a syringe and tube. The drain is placed, the syringe attached and the plunger withdrawn to achieve the desired negative pressure. A pin is placed through the plunger to secure it in place.

TYPE OF IMPLANT

The following types of drain are available:

- Surface-acting drains: Penrose drains, corrugated drains
- Tube drains (single lumen)
- Sump drains (multi-lumen)
- Sump–Penrose drains (multi-lumen).

Penrose drains

This is a flattened, cylindrical, soft latex rubber tube (Figure 6.2). Sizes range from 0.5 to 5 cm wide, and from 30 to 90 cm long. This is a passive drain, which functions primarily by capillary action and gravity flow, and must be placed with its exit in a dependent position. Some fluid will exit via the lumen, particularly immediately following placement, but the majority of the fluid passes extraluminally over the surface of the drain. Fenestration of Penrose drains reduces their surface area, and hence their efficiency, and

should not be done. The Penrose drain is not suitable for use as an active drain since the negative pressure will cause the drain to collapse.

A *strip drain* is a thin strip of latex cut from a quarter-inch diameter Penrose drain. This is used as a narrow flat drain when an entire drain would be too wide.

Penrose drains are soft, easily sterilized and readily available. They are malleable and do not exert pressure on adjacent structures. They are readily tolerated by most patients. However, latex and other types of rubber incite more tissue reaction than silicone rubber or polypropylene drains and cause more rapid formation of a fibrous tract. This makes this type of drain more suitable for drainage of abscesses, where a sinus tract may be desirable.

Common mistakes in placing Penrose drains are making the skin exit wound too small, or tunnelling the drain too far subcutaneously before entering the wound, both of which result in an inadequate opening for fluid passage.

Corrugated drains

These are ribbed, malleable strips of rubber or PVC (see Figure 6.3). They have no internal lumen and drainage only occurs over their surface. Like all passive drains, their efficacy is dictated by their surface area. These drains are more rigid than Penrose drains and have the potential to cause more tissue irritation. A variant of this drain, the *Yeates tissue drain*, consists of a series of small tubes attached together in a flat sheet. This will drain both over its external surface and via the lumina.

Tube drains

These are cylindrical tubes with at least one lumen and may function as either passive or active drains (Figure 6.7). They may be constructed of rubber, silicone rubber, PVC, polyethylene or other plastics. Sizes range from 3½ to 40 French (1–13 mm internal diameter). As passive drains they remove fluid intraluminally by gravity, with a small amount extraluminally. As active drains they remove fluid exclusively by the internal lumen. To avoid collapse of the drain when suction is applied, they

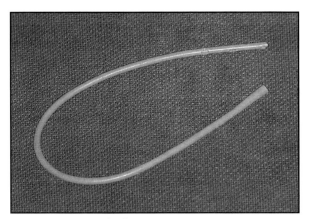

Figure 6.7: *Latex tube drain.*

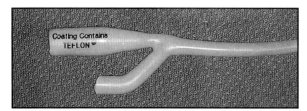

Figure 6.8: *Foley catheter with syringe adapter removed.*

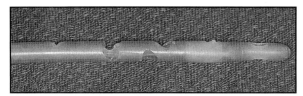

Figure 6.9: *Foley catheter fenestrated at tip.*

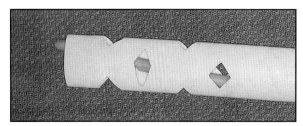

Figure 6.10: *Sump–Penrose drain.*

are manufactured from more rigid materials than are passive drains. Hence, they are more likely to cause tissue irritation and patient discomfort.

The section of drain within the wound needs to be fenestrated to increase the efficiency of fluid egress and to reduce the likelihood of obstruction by tissue or exudate. Fenestrations may be cut into a non-fenestrated tube. They should be oval, and should not occupy more than one third of the circumference of the tube to avoid kinking or breakage.

Potential disadvantages include occlusion of the lumen and collapse on applying suction. Red rubber tubes are more irritant to tissues than any other drains, whereas a minimal response occurs with silicone rubber tubes. An impurity in certain polyethylene tubes has been demonstrated to support bacterial growth.

Sump drains

These are tube drains with two or more lumina. The larger primary lumen provides the egress channel from the wound, while the smaller secondary lumen acts as a vent for access and circulation of air into the wound. This venting action reduces the likelihood of tube occlusion and increases the efficiency of drainage by displacing fluid from the wound. In general, the more lumina, the greater the efficacy of the drain.

Sump drains are available commercially or may be made from a Foley catheter. The syringe adapter is cut off (Figure 6.8) and the catheter is fenestrated at the tip (Figure 6.9). Air is allowed into the wound by removing the inflatable bulb or ensuring the fenestrations encroach on the bulb inflation channel. The wider, central channel acts as the egress, and the smaller inflation channel allows venting. The main disadvantage is the possibility of contamination of the wound via the ingress channel. For this reason this portal should be fitted with a bacterial filter.

Sump–Penrose drain

This is a triple-lumen drain created by placing a double-lumen sump drain inside a Penrose drain (Figure 6.10). The Penrose drain may be fenestrated,

and gauze padding may be incorporated between the Penrose drain and the sump drain to increase the efficiency of capillary action and to reduce tissue trauma by the more rigid sump drain. The Penrose drain is attached by encircling sutures at either end.

The advantage is that the outer fenestrated Penrose drain allows fluid to exit while preventing tissue adherence to the sump drain. This design allows the drains to remain functional in tissues for long periods. These drains were initially designed for intra-abdominal drainage but have now been superseded by the technique of open peritoneal drainage.

A *modified sump–Penrose drain* contains another tube within the Penrose drain. These are available commercially, or may be made by adding a rubber urethral catheter to the Penrose–Foley catheter outlined above. The presence of three lumina allows suction to be applied to one lumen, an irrigating fluid to be introduced via the second, and air to enter via the third.

DRAIN PLACEMENT AND MANAGEMENT

The following general guidelines apply to drain placement and management:

• Drains should be manufactured from soft, inert radiopaque materials which induce minimal tissue reaction

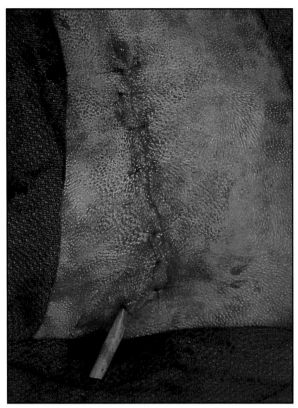

Figure 6.11: *Penrose drain exiting dependently, away from sutured wound.*

- Drains should not exit through the primary incision or make contact with the suture line as this will interfere with healing (Figure 6.11)
- Drains should not be placed near major neurovascular bundles or anastomotic sites, since they may cause erosion of these structures
- Sutures placed to close the wound should be placed carefully to avoid incorporating the drain
- For surface-acting drains, the exit holes should be of a sufficient size to allow adequate drainage, but not so large as to risk herniation of tissue from the wound. For a Penrose drain, this is approximately 1.5 to 2 times the diameter of the drain
- For passive drains exit holes must be gravitationally dependent
- The minimum effective number of exit holes should be used, which should be dependent if using passive drains
- A large area of hair should be clipped around the wound, particularly dependently
- Petroleum-based jelly may be applied beneath the exit hole to prevent excoriation, but should not occlude the hole
- Drain placement should allow aseptic postoperative care
- The protruding drain and the exit holes should be cleaned at least twice daily to avoid obstruction and to reduce the risk of ascending infection

- A sterile dressing and a light bandage should be applied and changed as often as required to maintain asepsis
- The suction device should be changed as often as required to maintain suction.

The Penrose drain should be placed into the wound before closure via a separate, dependent stab incision:

- A pair of haemostatic forceps is used to create a tunnel between the ventral aspect of the wound and a point just beneath the skin ventral to this. A stab incision is made over the forceps and the forceps used to grasp the drain and pull it into the wound (Figure 6.12a)
- The drain should be anchored proximally within the wound with a single absorbable suture. As small a bite as possible is taken of the drain so that it will easily tear through on removal (Figure 6.12b)
- Alternatively, the proximal end of the drain may be anchored to the skin with a monofilament suture passed through the skin and through the drain (Figure 6.12c). The suture is then passed back out through the skin and tied externally
- The drain should be cut so that only 1–2 cm protrudes beyond the skin. This end is then anchored to the skin with a single monofilament suture (Figure 6.12d).

The drain may also be placed with separate stab incisions above and below the wound and be anchored to the skin at each point (Figure 6.12e). However, there will be no effective drainage from the non-dependent exit hole and this technique increases the likelihood of wound contamination, and should be avoided.

Tube drains are also placed prior to closure via a separate stab incision. All of the fenestrated part of the drain should lie within the wound. Commercially available tube drains may have a trochar at the non-fenestrated end to allow atraumatic passage of the drain from wound to external skin surface (Figure 6.13). A tube drain may be placed into a wound that has already been closed or into a wound cavity using a trochar in the drain or using the Seldinger guide wire technique.

Tube drains are not usually anchored within the wound and therefore secure fixation to the skin at the exit hole needs to be achieved. A Chinese finger trap friction suture or a tape butterfly sutured to the skin may be used. If suction is to be applied to the drain, then an airtight seal is required at all points of the wound. Routine primary closure and the resulting fibrin seal may be adequate in most cases, although this can be augmented by the judicious application of topical antibiotic ointment (Pavletic, 1993).

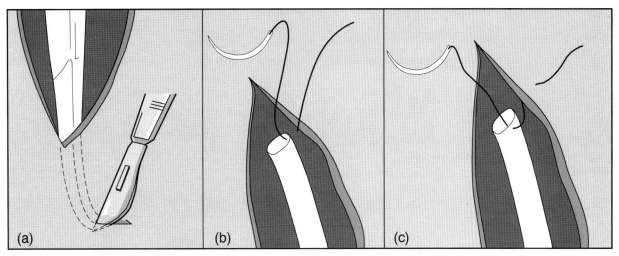

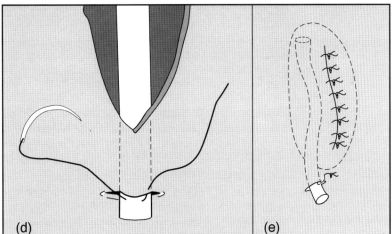

Figure 6.12: *Penrose drain placement. (a) Stab incision over tip of haemostats tunnelled subcutaneously from the wound. (b) Drain anchored internally by simple interrupted absorbable suture placed through wound tissue and edge of drain. (c) Drain anchored externally by simple interrupted non-absorbable suture placed through skin and drain. The suture is then passed back out through the skin and tied externally. (d) Distal end of drain anchored to skin with simple interrupted non-absorbable suture. (e) Single exit drain, anchored to the skin distally.*

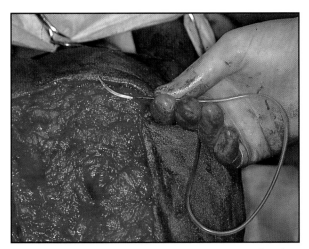

Figure 6.13: *Trochar used for atraumatic passage of a tube drain.*

DRAIN REMOVAL

As a guideline, a drain should be left *in situ* until the drainage subsides. The drain should be inspected regularly and the amount of fluid in the reservoir or the dressing noted. All drains incite a foreign body reaction which results in the production of fluid.

Hence there will always be some fluid at the exit port of any drain; this may be up to 50 ml/day in a large wound. Drains should be removed as soon as possible to reduce the possibility of wound contamination and the development of a sinus tract, which will generally take 3–5 days.

Drains placed in small potential cavities to evacuate capillary bleeding may usually be removed in 24 hours. Drains placed to evacuate exudate from a site of bacterial infection may need to be left for 2–3 days. Drains placed to facilitate union of tissues, such as after excision of large masses, should be removed once the dead space has been obliterated. This may take 5–10 days, although occasionally longer periods of up to 2–3 weeks may be required. Prolonged wound drainage is common in traumatic wounds with extensive muscle trauma (e.g. dog bites) and in elbow hygromas. In most patients, the drain should be removed when the fluid diminishes to a small con-sistent volume and is serosanguinous in consistency.

The drain is removed by first cutting the suture that anchors the drain to the skin. In the case of a Penrose drain, where a suture retains the drain within the wound, the drain is removed with a sharp downward tug.

If both ends of the drain exit the wound:

1. The first suture is removed
2. The drain is stretched and cut at a section which lay in the wound
3. The second suture is cut and the remainder of the drain removed.

Immediately after removal, the drain should be inspected to ensure that none has been left behind in the wound. The exit hole is left to heal by second intention.

COMPLICATIONS

It is important to realize that drains are not benign. If used incorrectly, the complications associated with drain placement may be more serious than the problem they were used to treat.

Wound infection

Drain placement increases the risk of wound infection. The physical presence of the drain will result in impairment of the local tissue resistance to bacterial infection because of the foreign body reaction, pressure ischaemia and tissue adhesion breakdown at drain removal. The presence of an exit hole increases the likelihood of bacteria gaining access to the wound. The infection rate increases directly with the duration of drainage. The infection rate also depends on the type and technique of drainage. A survey of 18,045 clean surgical wounds showed that drainage increased the infection rate and that this was higher with passive drains than with closed suction drains (Figure 6.14) (Cruse, 1973).

This complication is minimized by strict asepsis when placing and managing the drain. A large area of skin should be clipped surrounding the drain and a sterile dressing may be of benefit. The fewest number and smallest diameter drains compatible with good drainage should be selected. They should be placed judiciously to prevent motion of the drain, and should be left in situ for the minimum length of time.

Type of drainage	Infection rate
Undrained	1.53%
Closed suction	1.8%
Penrose drain (separate stab incision)	2.4%
Penrose drain (through primary incision)	4%

Figure 6.14: Influence of drains on wound infection rate. (Data from Cruse, 1973.)

Wound dehiscence

There is an increased risk of incisional dehiscence and herniation of tissues if drains exit through the primary wound, or if large exit holes are made. Drains should be placed through a separate stab incision, which should be as small as possible whilst still being compatible with good drainage.

Premature loss or retention

Inadequate fixation of the drain may result in the drain falling out, or being easily removed by the patient. The presence of strong adhesions in the wound, a large bite of drain incorporated in an anchoring suture, or large fenestrations in the drain may cause the drain to fragment in the wound.

The number, size and length of any drains placed should always be noted in the patient's record. Drains should be fixed securely in place and suitable measures taken to prevent the patient from interfering with the drains, e.g. Elizabethan collar or bandage. Radiopaque drains allow their detection if they are retained within a wound.

Failure of drainage

This can usually be traced to one of the following:

- Improper drain placement
- Use of a tube of inadequate diameter
- Loss of negative pressure in the suction system because of detachment or overfilling of the reservoir
- Obstruction of the drain.

In most cases a loss of negative pressure can be corrected by re-attaching another reservoir, or evacuating the one attached.

A tube drain may be obstructed by tissue or discharge. It may be possible to relieve such an obstruction by flushing with a small volume of sterile irrigating fluid. However, this introduces the potential for contamination and should be avoided. If the drain is already in a contaminated or infected wound (e.g. an abscess) and drainage is essential, then flushing may be justified. Otherwise the drain should be removed. Another drain should be inserted if continued drainage is required. The use of a fenestrated drain reduces the likelihood of this complication.

Pain and irritation

The presence of drains will cause some irritation and pain, and may be responsible for an elevated temperature postoperatively. This may cause the patient to remove the drain or to mutilate the wound. Suitable restraint devices and adequate analgesia should be provided at all times.

Drain tract cellulitis

This is a minor but common problem. Clinical signs include erythema, induration and pain at the exit site. The likelihood and severity of the inflammation increases the longer the drain is left in the wound. This problem generally resolves on removing the drain.

Misuse and over-reliance

The surgeon should not rely on the drain to compensate for improper intraoperative or postoperative management. Drains cannot substitute for proper haemostasis, gentle tissue handling and adequate debridement and lavage. Drains may tempt a surgeon to close a wound that would be better left open.

PRACTICAL CONSIDERATIONS

Although many drainage systems are available, the practical choices in most cases are much simpler. The most commonly used drains in wound management are the Penrose drain and the closed suction tube drain. Although the commercially available closed suction units are more expensive than Penrose drains, this additional cost is relatively small when considering the large investment in terms of medical care and surgery already made on behalf of the patient, and the reduced morbidity. This cost may be reduced if a 'home-made' suction device is constructed.

Specific applications

Subcutaneous drainage (e.g. in traumatic wounds, abscesses, wounds with dead space following large mass removal, elbow hygroma) can be achieved with simple drains such as a Penrose drain. Deep pocket wounds may be drained with either a Penrose drain or a closed suction drain, the advantages of the latter making them more useful.

Adequate drainage is critical to the survival of skin flaps and grafts. Haematoma and seroma formation under free skin grafts is the most common cause of their failure (Pavletic, 1993). The most effective technique for removing fluid from full thickness free skin grafts is continuous closed suction (Pope and Swaim, 1986). The other techniques, in decreasing order of effectiveness, are: an expanded meshed graft; a non-expanded meshed graft; and multiple parallel rows of stab incisions ('pie crust' incisions).

Practical recommendations would be to use 'pie crust' incisions in a free skin graft (see Chapter 9) and

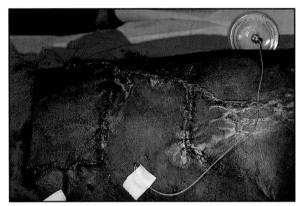

Figure 6.15: *Closed suction tube drain placed after wound reconstruction with skin flaps.*

Copyright © R.A.S. White.

to use a closed suction drain under a skin flap (Figure 6.15). This drain should be secured to prevent it moving beneath the flap and interfering with adhesion and should exit at a point away from the pedicle to preserve the blood supply.

REFERENCES AND FURTHER READING

Cruse PJE (1973) A five year prospective study of 23,649 surgical wounds. *Archives of Surgery* **107,** 206–210

Donner GS and Ellison GW (1986) The use and misuse of abdominal drains in small animal surgery. *Compendium of Continuing Education* **8,** 705–712

Fox S (1988) The best methods of wound drainage in pets. *Veterinary Medicine* **83,** 462–472

Hampel N (1993) Surgical drains. In: *Surgical Complications and Wound Healing in the Small Animal Practice*, ed. J. Harari, pp.319–347. WB Saunders, Philadelphia

Hosgood G (1990) The history of surgical drainage. *Journal of the American Veterinary Medical Association* **196,** 42–44

Lee AH, Swaim SF and Henderson RA (1986) Surgical drainage. *Compendium of Continuing Education* **8,** 94–103

Pavletic (1993) *Atlas of Small Animal Reconstructive Surgery.* JB Lippincott, Philadelphia

Pope ER and Swaim S (1986) Wound drainage from under full thickness skin grafts in dogs. I: Quantitative evaluation of four techniques. *Veterinary Surgery* **15,** 65–71

Swaim SF and Henderson RA (1997) *Small Animal Wound Management, 2nd edn.* Williams and Wilkins, Baltimore

Swaim SF and Lee AH (1990) Wound drainage techniques. In: *Current Techniques in Small Animal Surgery*, ed. MJ Bojrab, pp.29–33. Lea and Febiger, Philadelphia

Williams JM, McHugh D and White RAS (1992) Use of drains in small animal surgery. *In Practice* **14,** 73–81

CHAPTER SEVEN

Tension Relieving Techniques and Local Skin Flaps

David Fowler

INTRODUCTION

The elasticity of skin and, therefore, the ease with which large wounds may be reconstructed varies tremendously among species. Dogs and cats have highly elastic skin, which minimizes the difficulty of managing tensile forces affecting wounds. The free mobility of canine and feline skin is attributed to two factors. First, skin in these species is nourished by cutaneous arteries which supply relatively large regions of skin. Skin, therefore, can be moved freely on underlying tissues without compromising its vascular supply. Secondly, dogs and cats have a well developed system of cutaneous musculature, consisting of the platysma muscle (head and neck) and the cutaneous trunci muscle (thorax and abdomen). Cutaneous vasculature courses deep to this musculature, which is free of deep fascial attachments.

Intact skin is normally under the influence of tensile forces, and dermal collagen is remodelled accordingly. This is intuitively obvious because skin, when incised, retracts to form a gap. The magnitude of tensile forces, as well as their direction, varies according to location. Tension lines have been described previously and are orientated in a direction similar to the stripes on a zebra. The direction of maximum tension is easily determined by pinching folds of skin in multiple planes to see which offers the least resistance (Figure 7.1). The direction in which skin is most easily moved is termed the line of maximum distensibility and is usually perpendicular to the line of maximum tension.

Excessive tensile forces acting on wounds pose several problems for the surgeon:

- Direct wound closure may prove impossible if forces are of sufficient magnitude
- Excessive tension during wound closure may embarrass blood flow through surrounding skin, increasing the risk of incisional dehiscence
- Restricted movement and postoperative pain may be seen, especially in wounds situated near flexor or extensor surfaces
- Excessively taut closure of extremity wounds can cause a tourniquet effect, resulting in oedema or disruption of vascular flow to the distal limb (Figure 7.2).

Tension can result in hypertrophic scar formation, although this is of greater concern in people than in dogs and cats.

Surgical techniques that utilize local tissues for the management of tensile forces during wound closure include undermining of surrounding skin, walking sutures to redistribute tension throughout the wound, incisional 'plasties' designed to redistribute tension in alternative directions, and local (random pattern or subdermal plexus) skin flaps used to move tissues from areas of relative excess into areas of relative need.

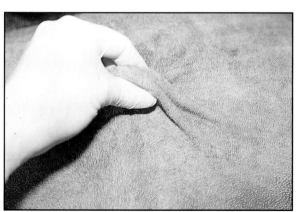

Figure 7.1: The elasticity of skin in different planes can be assessed by pinching skin folds in various directions.

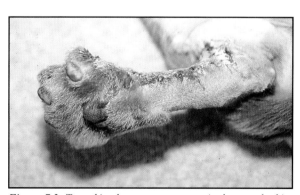

Figure 7.2: Taut skin closure on an extremity has resulted in compromise of venous and lymphatic drainage, and swelling of the foot, in this cat with a metatarsal injury. Release of the closure is required to prevent secondary injury to distal tissues.

The decision as to which procedure is best depends on multiple factors, including location of the wound, regional availability of skin, magnitude of tensile forces or distensibility surrounding the wound, risk of delayed closure and preference of the surgeon. In general, the simplest and most cost-effective techniques should be used. However, it is important to identify in advance wounds that will benefit from more advanced or aggressive reconstructive techniques. Examples might include traumatic soft tissue wounds associated with open fractures or extensive oncological resections.

PATTERNS OF WOUND CLOSURE

Simple side-to-side closure is frequently not the most efficient or cosmetic method of wound reconstruction. Determining the ideal pattern of wound closure depends on assessing the magnitude and direction of planes of tension and distensibility surrounding the wound, as well as the shape of the defect. Wounds should be closed with the least tension and the best cosmetic appearance possible.

Managing 'dog-ears'

The term dog-ear refers to a bunching of tissue at the ends of a wound. Dog-ears are formed when fusiform defects with sides of unequal length are closed, or when wounds with a small length:width ratio are sutured side-to-side. Small dog-ears are frequently ignored, and resolve as redistribution of wound tension occurs over time. Larger dog-ears should be addressed at the time of wound reconstruction to provide a cosmetic closure. Many techniques have been described for the elimination or prevention of dog-ears:

- Dog-ear formation can be minimized by distributing length discrepancies between unequal sides of a fusiform defect throughout the suture line (Figure 7.3). This is most easily accomplished by first placing a suture at the mid-point of both sides, resulting in the formation of two smaller defects with unequal sides. Additional sutures are placed at the mid-points of each of these defects. Suturing continues until the defect is closed. By suturing in this fashion the length discrepancy between sides is distributed throughout the suture line rather than concentrated at one end.
- Larger dog-ears are more easily managed by excision (Figure 7.4). The simplest technique involves elevation of the dog-ear to form a triangular shape. Sharp incision is made through the skin on either side of the base of the triangle and the resulting defect is closed routinely.

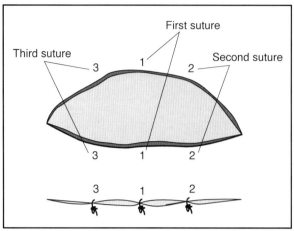

Figure 7.3: Tissue should be distributed evenly when closing ovoid excisions with unequal margins. This is accomplished by first placing a single suture at the mid-point of both sides. Remaining defects are closed by sequential placement of further 'dividing' sutures.

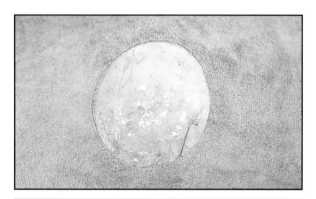

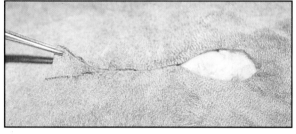

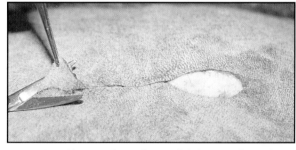

Figure 7.4: Closure of round or oval defects results in the formation of triangular 'dog-ears'. When excess tissue is available, dog-ears are most easily managed by simple excision of the redundant tissue.

Circular and ovoid wounds

Various techniques facilitate the cosmetic closure of circular defects (Swaim and Henderson, 1997). The technique of choice depends primarily on the amount of redundant skin surrounding the defect:

- Direct closure of circular defects results in the formation of large dog-ears. This can be prevented by excising triangular pieces of skin from opposing ends of the defect, thereby converting a circular defect into a fusiform defect with a 4:1 length:width ratio (Figure 7.5). Skin surrounding the wound should be manipulated to determine the lines of greatest and least tension, and skin excision should be performed such that the resulting fusiform defect is orientated parallel to the line of greatest tension.

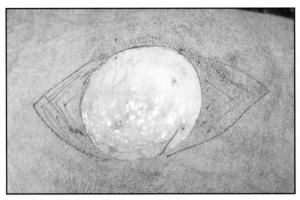

Figure 7.5: Dog-ear formation can be avoided by converting round or ovoid excisions into fusiform excisions with a 4:1 length:width ratio. The shaded area indicates tissue to be excised. This technique is useful in areas with redundant or elastic skin.

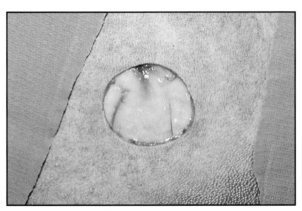

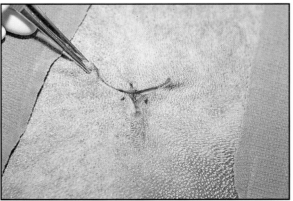

Figure 7.6: In areas with minimal skin elasticity, dog-ear formation can be minimized by triangulating the closure of round defects. Small dog-ears formed at the ends of each arm of the closure can be excised.

- The amount of tissue that needs to be excised to ensure a cosmetic closure can be reduced by performing a three-point closure of circular defects (Figure 7.6). A single subcutaneous or intradermal suture is placed into three equidistant points and tied, thereby converting the circular defect into three smaller fusiform defects. Dog-ears will be formed at the ends of all three fusiform defects; they should be sutured as described previously.

- When little or no elastic or redundant skin is available for reconstruction, a combined V closure should be considered (Figure 7.7). V-shaped incisions are made at opposing sides of the circular defect such that the arms of the V form two sides of an equilateral triangle pointing toward the centre of the defect. The height of this imaginary equilateral triangle equals the radius of the defect. Following incision, the flaps are undermined and transposed within the defect. The tips of the flaps are sutured such that five smaller fusiform defects result, all of which have roughly equal sides. Continued routine closure results in an irregularly shaped suture line with minimal dog-ear formation.

Square, rectangular and triangular wounds

Square, rectangular and triangular defects are most easily closed using a technique of centripetal closure (Figure 7.8). Subcutaneous or intradermal closure begins at the four corners of the defect. Tissues are progressively apposed until all suture lines converge. When dealing with square defects, all four suture lines will converge at the centre of the defect. In rectangular defects, suture lines at opposing ends of the rectangle will converge with each other and the remaining defect is closed side-to-side in a routine manner. Dehiscence is not uncommon at the junction of multiple suture lines. Tissues in these regions should be manipulated with care, and sutures placed precisely to minimize vascular disruption.

MOBILIZATION TECHNIQUES

Direct closure techniques are often inadequate when dealing with large wounds, or wounds located in areas with little redundant skin. By using techniques that capitalize on the viscoelastic properties of skin, however, the surgeon is often able to achieve wound closure without resorting to more advanced reconstructive options, such as skin flaps or skin grafts. Options to enhance mobilization of skin include undermining, walking sutures, presuturing, multiple punctate relaxing incisions and acute or subacute skin expansion.

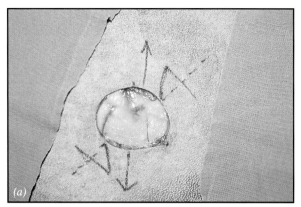

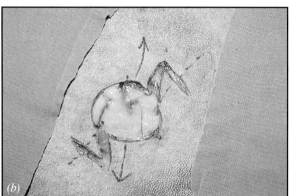

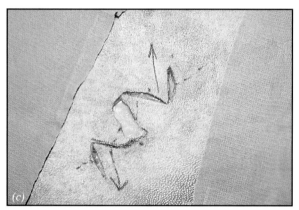

Figure 7.7: *Combined V closure can be used in areas with little or no elastic skin surrounding a round excision. (a) The arms of the V to be incised are indicated. Arrows indicate the direction of maximal tension. (b) The arms of the V have been incised. (c) Undermining and transposition of the flaps results in a redistribution of tension.*

Undermining

Undermining skin surrounding a wound is one of the simplest and most effective methods of reducing tension during wound closure. Loose connective tissue attachments are severed between the skin and deeper tissues, thereby facilitating cutaneous advancement over the wound. Extensive undermining should be performed deep to cutaneous musculature, in areas where such exists, to preserve the vascular integrity of the skin.

There is no absolute formula to determine the extent to which surrounding tissue must be undermined. The directions of tensile forces acting on the wound are first determined by grasping and manipulat-

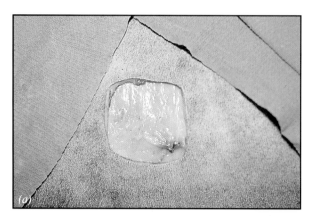

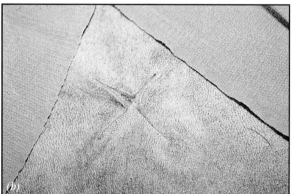

Figure 7.8: *Square or rectangular defects are most easily closed using a centripetal closure beginning at each corner of the defect and extending toward the centre.*

ing surrounding skin. Skin is then undermined parallel to the proposed direction of advancement (Figure 7.9). Skin edges are periodically assessed for ease of advancement over the wound and undermining is discontinued when opposing skin margins are brought into apposition with minimal tension.

Undermining, while reducing tension and facilitating wound closure, also increases wound dead space. In most instances, drains should be used for dead space management after extensive tissue undermining. Either passive latex drains or active closed-suction drains can be used successfully. Drains may be unnecessary in locations where the application of a bandage assists in maintaining apposition of tissue planes and in reducing shearing forces acting upon tissue layers within the wound.

Walking sutures

Walking sutures have a two-fold purpose:

- They serve to obliterate dead space after undermining and distribute tensile forces throughout the wound surface, as opposed to concentrating forces at the skin margins
- They facilitate the progressive advancement of undermined skin into the wound defect.

Initial sutures are placed between the dermis, at the deepest portions of undermined skin, and fascia within

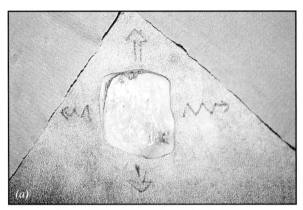 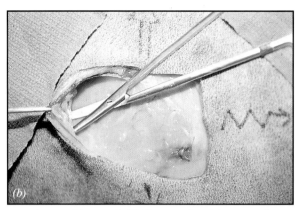

Figure 7.9: (a) Open arrows indicate the direction of maximal tension acting on this wound. (b) Tissue undermining is used to facilitate skin advancement over the defect. Tissue is undermined parallel to the direction of anticipated skin advancement.

the wound bed relatively nearer its centre (Figure 7.10). Proper suture placement into the dermis is confirmed by the formation of a dimple when the suture is tied or placed under tension. As the suture is tied, the 'base' of the undermined skin is advanced slightly towards the wound's centre. A second tier of walking sutures is then placed to provide further tissue advancement. Each tier of walking sutures thereby serves progressively to advance the skin edge toward the centre of the defect. Skin margins should lie in close apposition, with little tension, after completing the placement of walking sutures.

Walking sutures have two significant disadvantages:

- When used for closure of clean-contaminated wounds, the incidence of infection may be increased due to the multiple ischaemic foci formed and the quantity of foreign material placed within the wound
- Walking sutures may also compromise cosmetic appearance and increase postoperative pain due to the fixation of normally moveable skin to relatively immobile underlying fascia. Because of these sequelae, the author only uses this technique to achieve wound closure if it is absolutely necessary.

Presuturing

Presuturing is a means of mobilizing tissue in instances where advanced planning is feasible, such as surgical removal of a large lesion. This technique utilizes the properties of cutaneous viscoelasticity and mechanical creep to facilitate subsequent wound closure.

Plicating sutures are placed across the proposed area of excision 8–24 hours prior to surgery. Immediately prior to surgery, the sutures are removed and the lesion is excised. Subsequent closure is achieved with less tension and a reduced incidence of tissue strangulation and dehiscence.

Skin stretching is similar to presuturing in principle, but is used after the formation of an open wound. Skin stretchers consist of externally applied

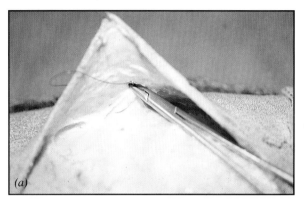

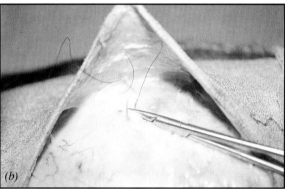

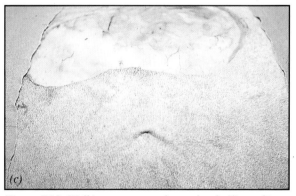

Figure 7.10: Walking sutures can be used to facilitate skin advancement and to distribute tensile forces over a large surface area. (a) Skin is first undermined and a suture bite is taken into the dermis at the deep margin of undermined skin. (b) A second bite is taken into fascia, relatively closer to the wound's centre. (c) Tying this suture advances the dermis to the point of fascial fixation. A 'dimple' is formed in the skin when a suture is placed at an appropriate depth into the dermis.

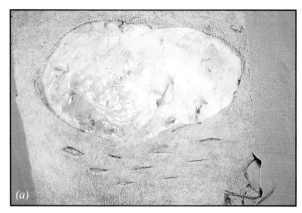 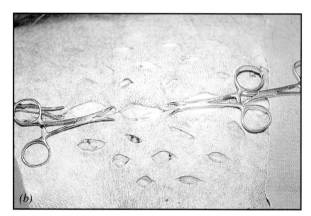

Figure 7.11: *Mesh expansion is used to facilitate skin advancement over large open wounds. (a) Staggered parallel rows of 1–2 cm incisions are made on either side of the defect. (b) As skin is advanced, the small incisions expand, resulting in the formation of many small open wounds. Second intention healing of these smaller wounds progresses at a much more rapid rate than does second intention healing of a single large wound.*

adhesive 'hook-pads' and elastic bands with a series of 'pile-pads' attached to their surface. The hook-pads are placed on either side of the wound and are connected under tension using the elastic bands. Tension is incrementally increased several times daily over a 2-4 day period until apposition of wound margins is achieved.

Multiple punctate relaxing incisions (mesh expansion)

Relaxing incisions are considered when, after under-mining skin surrounding the wound, tension continues to preclude direct closure. Staggered rows of punctate incisions are made, full thickness, through skin surrounding the defect, beginning nearest the wound margin (Figure 7.11). Incisions may vary but are normally 1-2 cm in length. Incisions should be separated by several centimetres to ensure that adequate blood supply is maintained to the elevated skin. Multiple staggered rows of incisions are made on either side of the wound.

As the skin margins are advanced to cover the wound, the punctate incisions form gaps, allowing the undermined skin to expand. The amount of skin expansion obtained is directly proportional to the length of the incisions and the number of incisions made. The multiple small open wounds created using this technique are bandaged and allowed to heal by contraction and epithelialization.

Skin expanders

There is very little literature describing the use of skin expanders in small animal surgery. Skin expanders consist of inflatable silastic chambers and are available in many different sizes and configurations. They are placed subcutaneously, adjacent to the wound bed, or adjacent to lesions prior to surgical excision. It is important to plan the location of the expander relative to the wound, since the expanded skin must subsequently be in a strategically advan-

tageous position for advancement or rotation over the defect. The incision for subcutaneous implantation of the expander also must be planned so that it is located at the leading edge of the advancement or rotation flap that will be formed at the time of wound reconstruction.

After implantation, the chamber is inflated over a course of days to weeks. Intraluminal pressure within the chamber is monitored and is maintained below normal capillary pressure. Expected tissue responses include epidermal hyperplasia, dermal collagen compression and the formation of granulation tissue and a fibrous capsule around the expander.

Skin expanders are associated with some problems:

- If pressures generated are too high, reduced vascular perfusion can cause necrosis of overlying skin
- Infection can occur, especially when expanders are used adjacent to contaminated wound beds
- Patient discomfort and pain during expansion has been reported in people, but has been difficult to evaluate in animals
- The fibrous capsule that forms around the tissue expander limits the pliability of overlying skin, making it difficult to mobilize over the wound
- Tissue expanders generally require staged reconstructive procedures separated by days to weeks, although acute intraoperative tissue expansion can be used to achieve an effect similar to presuturing.

REDISTRIBUTION OF TENSILE FORCES USING INCISIONAL 'PLASTIES'

V–Y plasty

The V–Y plasty is most commonly employed to correct functional consequences of wound contrac-

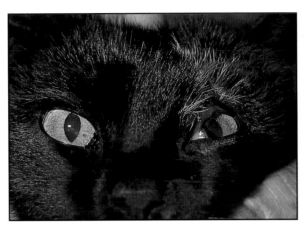

Figure 7.12: Previous cryosurgery has resulted in the formation of an iatrogenic ectropion in this cat. V–Y plasty can be used to reduce tensile forces on the upper lid.

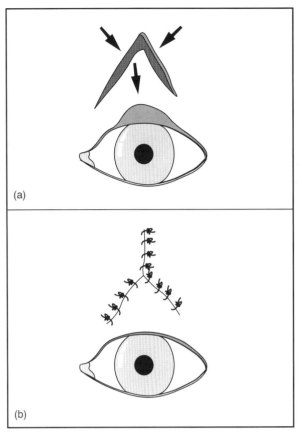

(a)

(b)

Figure 7.13: V–Y plasty is performed by converting a V-shaped incision into a Y-shaped closure. (a) The base of the V is situated at the leading edge of tissue advancement. Arrows indicate the direction of skin movement. (b) Side-to-side closure beginning at the apex of the V is performed until an adequate degree of tissue advancement is achieved. The arms of the resulting Y are then closed in a routine manner.

tion on normal structures adjacent to the wound. For example, wounds adjacent to the eyelid can result in the formation of an ectropion due to tensile forces placed on the eyelid during wound contraction (Figure 7.12). The goal of reconstruction in this situation is to reduce or redistribute these tensile forces, allowing the eyelid to assume a more functional position.

The V–Y plasty, in essence, is a single pedicle flap that is advanced towards its base rather than towards its apex (Figure 7.13):

1. The initial incision is in the form of a V, with the base of the flap oriented perpendicular to the line of tension and the vertex pointed opposite to the direction of movement
2. The V flap is undermined and the point of the resulting defect is closed side-to-side, forming the tail of a Y
3. Side-to-side suturing is continued until tissue advancement has adequately counteracted the pre-existing pathological tensile forces
4. The arms of the Y are then sutured routinely.

Flap advancement is achieved at the expense of increased tensile forces in a plane perpendicular to the direction of advancement. Therefore, it is important to ensure that increased tension in this plane will not result in additional adverse functional or cosmetic effects.

Z plasty

Z plasties are used to redistribute tension in opposing planes; a decrease in tension in one plane is achieved at the expense of increased tension in the opposite direction. They are most useful for the correction of wound contracture, a pathological state referring to a loss of function or mobility as a result of excessive wound contraction. A Z plasty may also be used as a relaxing incision to reorientate skin tension adjacent to an open wound.

The Z plasty is composed of a central limb and two arms, all of equal length (Figure 7.14). The lengths of the central limb and arms, as well as the angles formed between them, are directly proportional to the extent to which redistribution of tension occurs. Angles varying from 30 to 90 degrees can be used, but angles approximating 60 degrees are the most useful.

The Z plasty is formed such that the central arm of the Z is oriented parallel with the tension on the wound or scar. The triangular flaps created after incising the central limb and both arms are undermined and translocated, resulting in a reversal of the Z, and a reduction of tension in a plane parallel to the original central arm. This reduction of tension is achieved at the expense of increased tensile forces in the perpendicular plane. The tension relief provided by multiple Z plasties is additive. In situations where the lengths of the central limb and the arms are limited by regional anatomy, multiple Z plasties may be performed (Figure 7.15). Whether performing single or multiple Z plasties, it is important for the surgeon to manipulate the surrounding skin prior to surgery to determine if sufficient tissue is available for the redistribution of tension.

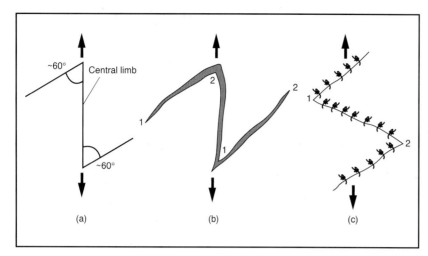

Figure 7.14: Z plasty is used for redistribution of tension in opposing directions. (a) The Z plasty consists of a central limb and two arms of equal length. The angles between the arms and the central limb approximate 60 degrees. Arrows indicate the line of maximum tension. (b) Incision is followed by undermining of the resulting triangular flaps. The flaps are then reversed. Numbers indicate points of suture placement. (c) Flap reversal results in the formation of a closure oriented in an opposite direction to that of the initial incision. Length has been gained in the direction of maximum tension, at the expense of increased tension in the opposing plane.

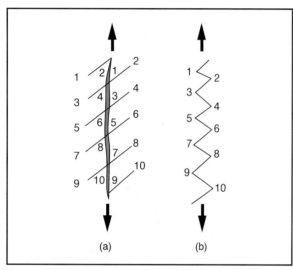

Figure 7.15: The effect of multiple Z plasties is additive. In situations where a long restrictive scar is present with little tissue in the opposing plane, multiple Z plasties can be considered. Arrows show the line of maximum tension. (a) Numbers indicate points of suture apposition. (b) Appearance of final reconstruction.

LOCAL FLAPS

Skin flaps are used to provide tissue to achieve closure of open wounds, or to redistribute tension away from wound margins. Flaps always maintain a vascular attachment at the donor site. Flaps are classified according to their vascular supply, the number and type of attachments maintained at the donor site, or the method by which they are moved from donor to recipient site.

They are termed 'axial pattern' or 'subdermal plexus (random pattern)' based on their vascular supply:

• Axial pattern flaps incorporate a direct cutaneous artery and vein in the flap design (see Chapter 8)
• Subdermal plexus flaps do not incorporate a direct cutaneous artery and vein and are dependent upon blood flow through the subdermal vascular plexus for nourishment.

The vascular integrity of subdermal plexus flaps is less consistent than is that of axial pattern flaps. Thus, the size of subdermal plexus flaps is limited and the base of attachment at the donor site must be relatively broad. It is difficult to make generalizations about safe length:width ratios for subdermal plexus flaps since this ratio varies according to factors such as anatomical site and wound tension. However, length:width ratios of 2:1 are generally considered quite safe; ratios exceeding 3:1 are at a progressively increasing risk of distal necrosis.

Deep sutures, such as walking sutures, should be avoided in the fixation of subdermal plexus flaps since they can compromise the vascular supply. Instead, subcutaneous or intradermal sutures are used to advance flaps and to distribute tension towards the base of the flap. Dead space can be managed with passive or active drains.

Flaps are termed single pedicle, double pedicle, or island, based on donor site attachment:

• Single pedicle flaps maintain one cutaneous donor site attachment
• Double pedicle flaps maintain two cutaneous donor site attachments
• In island flaps, all cutaneous attachments are transected, but a vascular attachment is maintained.

Subdermal plexus flaps are rarely dissected as island flaps due to the uncertainty of their vascular anatomy. Axial pattern flaps are routinely elevated as island flaps.

Flaps can be moved from donor to recipient site either directly or indirectly:

• Direct movement implies that the flap is elevated from the donor site and moved immediately into the recipient site
• Indirect movement implies staged procedures whereby the flap is moved progressively from donor to recipient site.

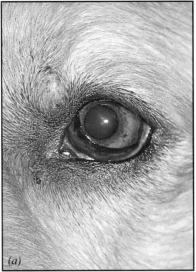
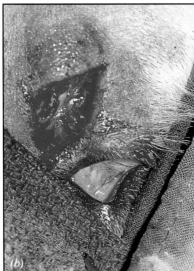
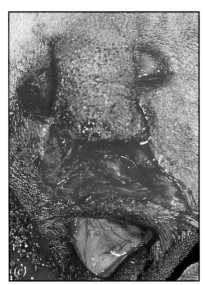
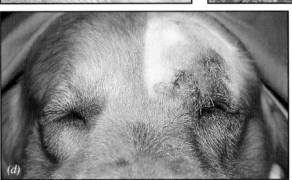

Figure 7.16: Single pedicle advancement flaps can be used to redistribute tension away from intolerant structures such as the eyelid. (a) This Golden Retriever presented with a 1 cm basal cell tumour located immediately adjacent to the upper eyelid margin. (b) Excision of the mass was performed, leaving a rectangular defect. (c) A single pedicle advancement flap was formed, extending distally from the eyelid margin. Burrow's triangles were excised on either side of the flap base to facilitate advancement without dog-ear formation. (d) Redistribution of tension away from the eyelid margin, and towards the base of the flap, has been accomplished with little or no resulting eyelid deformation.

Indirect flaps can be used when the donor site is too distant from the recipient site to allow direct movement of tissues into the defect. Indirect subdermal plexus flaps are rarely used currently, however, since alternatives such as axial pattern flaps, skin grafts and microvascular tissue transfer facilitate single-stage reconstruction of distant wounds. Direct subdermal plexus flaps are sub-classified as advancement, rotation or transposition flaps, according to the type of movement employed to reach the recipient wound bed.

Single pedicle advancement flaps

Single pedicle advancement flaps are used to facilitate closure of square or rectangular defects when tissue is available for closure only on one side of the wound (Figure 7.16). Examples include wounds near the eyelids or mouth.

1. The flap is created by extending parallel incisions from opposing edges of the wound
2. The long axis of the flap is oriented parallel to the direction of maximal skin distensibility
3. The resulting flap is undermined and is advanced directly into the wound bed, without changing the orientation of the donor site attachment
4. The leading corners of the advancement flap are sutured to the most distant corners of the wound defect

5. The remaining closure is performed side-to-side, thereby distributing tension along the length of the advancement flap.

Length:width ratios should be minimized, although larger length:width ratios are more effective at distributing tension and facilitating closure than are smaller ones. Delay procedures can be used if length:width ratios exceed 3:1 or if the surgeon is concerned about the vascular integrity of the flap. To perform a delay procedure, the flap is incised and undermined. The flap is not advanced into position, but rather is immediately sutured into its original position. Secondary flap elevation is performed after approximately 3 days, at which time the flap is advanced into the recipient site. Delay is of established benefit in extending flap survival, but carries the price of staged reconstruction and prolonged open wound management. As a general rule, alternative reconstructive procedures should be thoroughly considered prior to embarking on a staged reconstruction.

Dog-ears inevitably form at the base of advancement flaps. If small, these may be disregarded and expected to resolve with time. Larger dog-ears may be prevented by the excision of Burow's triangles at the base of the flap, prior to advancement:

1. Equilateral triangular pieces of skin are excised from either side of the flap

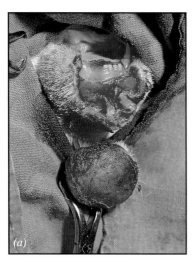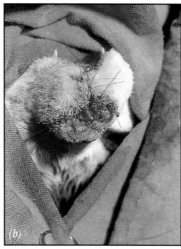

Figure 7.17: Bilateral single pedicle advancement flaps are used to close defects where tissue is available for advancement from either side of a tissue defect. (a) Excision of a tumour involving the upper lip has resulted in the formation of a full thickness lip defect in this cat. (b) Full thickness single pedicle advancement flaps have been formed from the lips bilaterally, and have been advanced to reconstruct the defect.

2. The side of the triangle should approximate the distance the flap is to be advanced
3. Excision of Burow's triangles must extend away from the base of the flap rather than into the base of the flap, since the latter will compromise blood supply.

Bilateral single pedicle advancement flaps

When tissue is available on opposing sides of the wound, single pedicle advancement flaps can be elevated and advanced from both sides, a technique also referred to as an H plasty (Figure 7.17). The principles discussed for single pedicle advancement flaps apply, with the exception that two opposing flaps are elevated and each is advanced to cover approximately half of the wound defect.

Bipedicle flaps

Bipedicle flaps maintain two cutaneous donor site attachments at opposing ends of the flap (Figure 7.18). This type of flap is used most often to facilitate wound closure on the extremities. Movement of the flap into the recipient site results in the formation of a secondary open wound. Tissue is, therefore, moved to cover critical structures such as exposed bone, and the secondary defect is planned so that it is situated over vascularized, non-compromised tissue such as muscle. The secondary defect can then be managed safely as an open wound, or can be reconstructed using alternative techniques such as full thickness skin grafts. The term 'single relaxing incision' is used to describe the formation of a bipedicle flap immediately adjacent to a wound.

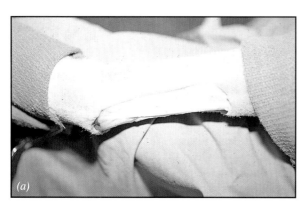

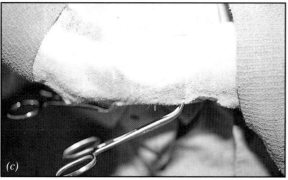

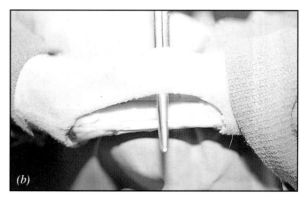

Figure 7.18: Bipedicle flaps are usually used to facilitate closure of wounds overlying critical structures such as exposed bones and nerves on the extremities. (a) An open wound is situated over the dorsal surface of the distal radius and carpus. (b) A full thickness skin incision has been made extending longitudinally along the palmar aspect of the radius. Abundant soft tissues are present in this location. The resulting skin flaps are undermined. (c) The skin flaps are advanced from either side to reconstruct the dorsal defect. The palmar defect is left to heal by second intention, or can be resurfaced using a skin graft.

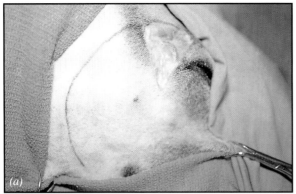

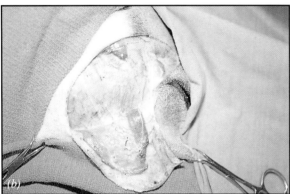

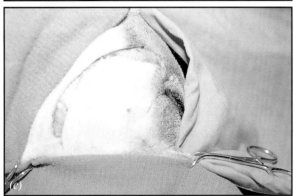

Figure 7.19: *Rotation flaps are used to redistribute tension away from intolerant structures such as the eyelid or prepuce. The length of incision should be approximately four times the distance of flap advancement.*

Rotation flaps

Rotation flaps are used for the reconstruction of triangular-shaped defects, particularly when direct reconstruction of the wound might distort critical structures such as the eyelid, prepuce or anus (Figure 7.19).

1. Tissues surrounding the wound are manipulated to determine from which direction the skin is most easily moved (i.e. where tension is least prevalent)
2. An arcuate, or semicircular, incision extending away from one side of the defect is created. As a general rule, the length of the incision should be approximately four times the distance the flap is to be moved
3. The entire flap is undermined deep to subcutaneous and superficial cutaneous muscle layers

4. The tip of the flap is advanced to the most distant point of the wound defect and sutured
5. Subcutaneous or intradermal sutures are placed to distribute tensile forces along the length of the incision and into the base of the flap.

Skin fold advancement flaps

Skin fold advancement flaps utilize redundant tissue in the axillary and inguinal skin folds for advancement into large wounds involving the pectoral and abdominal regions (Figure 7.20):

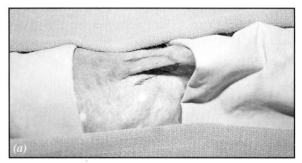

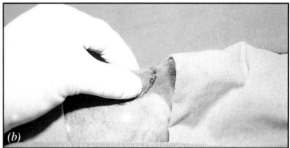

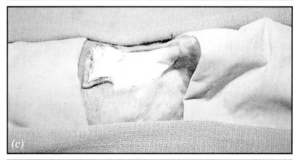

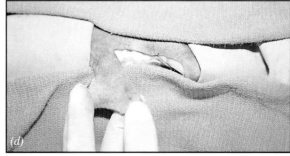

Figure 7.20: *Axial and inguinal skin fold flaps are useful for the reconstruction of large wounds involving adjacent sites. (a) The proposed incision is indicated. (b) The skin fold should be pinched to ensure that tension-free closure is possible following creation of the flap. (c, d) The resulting flap can be transposed on to the adjacent thoracic or abdominal wall.*

1. To form the skin flap, the axillary or inguinal skin fold is grasped between the surgeon's fingers and a level of incision is determined that will allow tension-free closure of the resulting defect

2. The base of the skin fold is incised from either side, beginning at the limb and extending towards the body. This results in the formation of a U-shaped skin flap with an attachment to the body wall

3. The donor site is closed using a direct side-to-side closure

4. The edges of the flap are unfolded and transposed to reconstruct adjacent defects.

Quite a large flap can be harvested safely using this technique without compromising limb function and range of motion.

REFERENCES AND FURTHER READING

Hunt GB (1995) Skin fold advancement flaps for closing large sternal and inguinal wounds in cats and dogs. *Veterinary Surgery* **24**, 172–174

Keller WG, Aron DN, Rakich PM, Crowe DT and Marks MA (1994) Rapid tissue expansion for the development of rotational skin flaps in the distal portion of the hindlimb of dogs: an experimental study. *Veterinary Surgery* **23**, 31–39

Madison JB, Donawick WJ, Johnston DE and Orsini RA (1989) The use of skin expansion to repair cosmetic defects in animals. *Veterinary Surgery* **18**, 15–21

Swaim SF and Henderson RA (1997) *Small Animal Wound Management*, 2ⁿᵈ edn. Williams & Wilkins, Baltimore

CHAPTER EIGHT

Axial Pattern Flaps

Audrey Remedios

INTRODUCTION

Large skin wounds, arising from trauma or surgical excision, can present reconstructive problems to the veterinary surgeon. The amount of local skin tension and the paucity of adjacent tissue may preclude primary closure of wounds, especially those involving the head, limbs and perineal regions. Other management options include second intention healing, tissue expanders, skin grafts and skin flaps. Second intention healing is associated with prolonged healing time and may result in a fragile epithelial surface and excessive wound contracture. Tissue expanders are implanted in the subcutaneous space and slowly expand the skin adjacent to a wound (Madison *et al.*, 1989). The redundant skin is then used to reconstruct the defect. Some disadvantages of expanders are implant cost, expander failure, and wound dehiscence and expander exposure. Free skin grafts are avascular and require optimal recipient beds and rapid revascularization for survival. Accordingly, traumatic wounds often require prolonged periods of open management prior to skin graft transfer. Skin flaps, which retain intact circulation from donor sites, are used in early wound reconstruction of suboptimal wound beds and are associated with fewer complications than second intention healing, tissue expanders or grafts.

BLOOD SUPPLY TO THE SKIN

In the dog and cat, the cutaneous circulation is connected to deep segmental vessels by direct cutaneous arteries and veins. These direct cutaneous vessels travel through intermuscular fascial septae and run parallel to the overlying skin at the subdermal level. Each direct cutaneous artery supplies an angiosome, or territory, composed of the superficial cutaneous musculature, subcutaneous tissue and skin (Figure 8.1).

The subdermal plexus is the major conduit of arterial supply to the skin. Where a layer of cutaneous muscle is present, the subdermal plexus lies both superficial and deep to it. In small animals, the major cutaneous muscles include the cutaneous trunci,

platysma, sphincter colli superficialis, prepucialis and supramammaricus muscles. Where the panniculus muscle is absent, such as in the middle and distal portions of the limbs, the subdermal plexus courses in the subcutaneous tissue on the deep face of the dermis. Branches from the subdermal plexus ascend to supply the dermis and epidermis. Thus, disruption of the subdermal plexus impairs circulation to the superficial skin layers.

CLASSIFICATION OF SKIN FLAPS

Skin flaps are classified according to blood supply as axial pattern or subdermal plexus. Axial pattern flaps are based on the angiosomes of direct cutaneous arteries and veins. All tissues within a defined

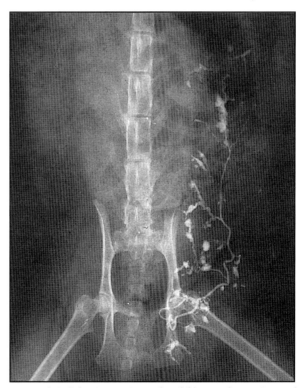

Figure 8.1: *Selective angiography of the vascular territory of the caudal superficial epigastric artery. This vessel supplies the glandular and subcutaneous tissue and skin of mammary glands 2, 3, 4 and 5 in the cat.*

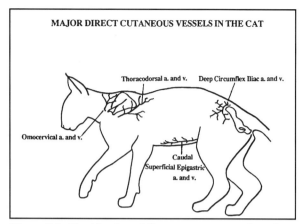

Figure 8.2: Identification of direct cutaneous vessels and their associated axial pattern flaps has been reported in the cat and dog. Such skin flaps can be used to reconstruct wounds involving the head and neck, the forelimb, the hindlimb and perineal regions.

vascular territory can be elevated from the body and will survive as long as the direct cutaneous vascular pedicle remains intact. Direct cutaneous arteries that sustain a large area of skin allow the development of axial pattern flaps of considerable length without vascular compromise. Subdermal plexus flaps are dependent upon terminal branches of the cutaneous circulation. As such, subdermal plexus flaps are limited in length when compared to axial pattern flaps. The mean survival area of axial pattern flaps is 50% greater than that of similarly sized subdermal plexus flaps.

AXIAL PATTERN SKIN FLAPS

Each axial pattern flap is based on the vascular territory supplied by distinct direct cutaneous vessels (Taylor and Palmer, 1987). These vessels and their angiosomes have been identified and mapped in the dog and cat (Figure 8.2). In general, the location of each vascular pedicle and the relative sizes of the supplied territories are similar in dogs and cats. However, the extremely pliable feline skin and similarity in body size and limb length facilitates more distal limb coverage provided by axial pattern flaps in cats than dogs.

Because axial pattern skin flaps have an excellent blood supply, they have several advantages over other methods of reconstruction:

- Axial pattern flaps can cover most large defects using one-stage procedures
- They have excellent survival rates, ranging from 96–100%
- Unlike free skin grafts, axial pattern flaps can be used to reconstruct indicated wounds associated with less than optimal conditions such as contamination, uneven surfaces or exposed bone, tendon and cartilage

- Early wound reconstruction without prolonged periods of open wound management is feasible
- The blood supply associated with axial pattern flaps minimizes the risk of postoperative infection. In instances of infection, overall flap survival is not adversely affected if treated with appropriate antibiotics (Trevor *et al.*, 1992)
- Axial pattern flaps are relatively simple to dissect and do not require specialized equipment.

There are some disadvantages associated with axial pattern flaps:

- Extensive surgical dissection of the donor bed is required for flap elevation
- Closure of the donor bed may require undermining and walking sutures to appose the surgically created defect
- The cosmetic appearance of the recipient area differs from that of the surrounding skin: characteristics such as hair direction, colour and length, glandular formation and the amount of subcutaneous fat are retained from the donor site (Figure 8.3).

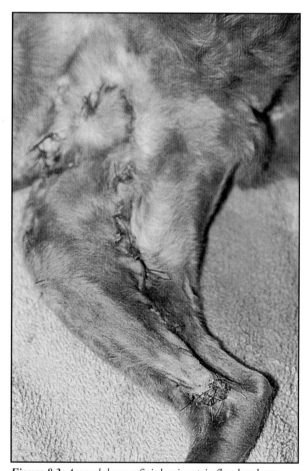

Figure 8.3: A caudal superficial epigastric flap has been rotated from the ventral abdomen to cover a distal tibial defect in a cat. This axial pattern flap is transferred with its associated mammary glands and subcutaneous fat. Direction of fur growth is different from the recipient bed.

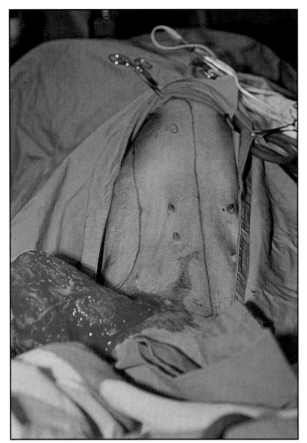

Figure 8.4: Prior to surgery, the limits of the caudal superficial epigastric flap are drawn on the skin with a felt-tipped marker.

Preoperative considerations

The cause and nature of a wound are important preoperative considerations that influence the appropriate time of closure. Surgically created defects, most commonly associated with tumour excision, are usually clean wounds. Because these wounds are uncontaminated and devoid of residual necrotic tissue, axial pattern flaps can be harvested and transferred directly on to the fresh wound bed. Traumatic wounds are contaminated or dirty, and are often associated with continued tissue necrosis for several days after injury. Such wounds often require several days of open management prior to delayed primary reconstruction using an axial pattern flap.

Adequate planning must be undertaken prior to dissection of axial pattern flaps. It is essential to know which flaps are most appropriate given the size, dimensions and location of the wound. The vascular limits of each flap determine the size and length of flap that can be harvested and transferred to an adjacent or distant location. Preoperatively, measurements should be taken to ensure the length and size of flap can reach and cover the wound. A smaller flap, less than total vascular flap territory, can be raised if dictated by the size and location of the wound. However, with large skin defects, all possible flap designs and methods of reconstruction should be considered.

For example, closure of a large wound involving the perineal area may require an axial pattern in conjunction with a subdermal plexus flap; coverage of an extensive limb wound may require both an axial pattern flap and skin graft. For distant skin wounds, an extended axial pattern flap that incorporates an adjacent angiosome can be harvested. Blood supply between the additional angiosome and the primary flap is maintained by anastomotic 'choke' vessels. These communications, however, are fragile, and survival of the entire extended flap is less predictable than the primary flap.

It is essential to know the following: the anatomical landmarks associated with the location of the vascular pedicle; the direction in which these vessels travel in relation to the underlying tissues; and the boundaries of vascular territory. A felt-tipped marker should be used preoperatively to delineate the anatomical location of the vascular pedicle and the limits of the flap (Figure 8.4). The patient must be positioned carefully prior to outlining the proposed flap, since skin distortion may alter the relationship of the skin to the underlying anatomical landmarks.

Axial pattern flaps can also be harvested as peninsular or island configurations. Peninsular axial pattern flaps are incised at each flap edge but retain a border of intact skin directly adjacent to the vascular pedicle (Figure 8.5). Mobility of the peninsular flap is decreased because of the skin attachment. Island axial pattern flaps have no cutaneous attachments and are connected to the donor bed only by the direct cutaneous artery and vein (Figure 8.6). The island configuration enhances flap mobility and prevents 'dog-ear' formation at the flap base. However, the vessels lose some protection from the overlying skin and may be kinked or placed under tension more easily during flap rotation. Island flaps and peninsular axial pattern flaps have similar survival areas.

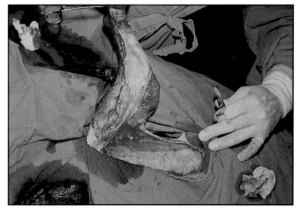

Figure 8.5: The peninsular axial pattern flap retains a border of intact skin directly adjacent to the vascular pedicle. This caudal superficial epigastric flap maintains connection to the skin in the area of the inguinal ring where the vacular pedicle emerges. Rotation of this flap distally is limited by the peninsular configuration.

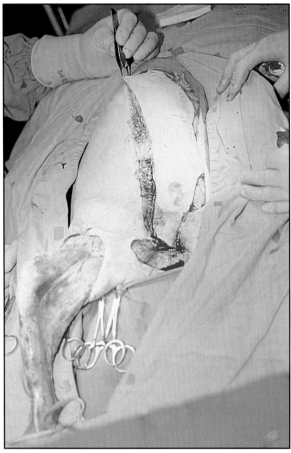

Figure 8.6: This caudal superficial epigastric flap is harvested in an island configuration and does not retain any cutaneous attachments. Although rotation of this flap is enhanced, care has to be taken to avoid kinking the vessels.

Flap dissection

This is done in the following way:

1. Dissection of an axial pattern flap begins with sharp incision of the flap borders followed by elevation of the flap

2. It is easiest and safest to establish the plane of dissection at the border furthest from the vascular pedicle. The level of surgical dissection should always be beneath the cutaneous muscle layer so as to preserve the subdermal plexus. In areas devoid of this muscle, such as the middle to distal limbs, dissection should be performed in the deep subcutaneous layer

3. Once the appropriate tissue plane is identified, elevation of the entire flap is performed, using sharp scissor dissection, towards the vascular pedicle. Haemostasis can be achieved using electrocautery. Upon approaching the direct cutaneous artery and vein, dissection must proceed cautiously to avoid inadvertent laceration of these vessels

4. The vascular pedicle does not have to be entirely exposed; rather, a surrounding cushion of subcutaneous fat can be left in place

5. The entire axial pattern flap is rotated to cover the wound. It is important that the vascular pedicle is not kinked or placed under tension during flap transfer and rotation. Flap rotation up to 180 degrees can be performed safely

6. Wounds that are located distant to the donor bed require a bridging excision of intact skin to connect the donor and recipient sites (Figure 8.7)

7. Prior to closure, passive or active drains are placed within the recipient bed

8. Subcutaneous tacking sutures are best avoided at the recipient site to prevent inadvertent impairment of the flap vasculature. Subcutaneous walking sutures are, however, useful to decrease dead space, diminish tension and appose the skin edges in the donor bed

9. The flap borders are sutured on to the recipient borders using several simple interrupted skin sutures to tack the flap into position. The remaining incision lines can be filled in rapidly using a series of simple continuous sutures or skin staples. The skin edges of the donor bed are closed routinely.

Postoperative considerations

The most common postoperative complications associated with axial pattern skin flaps are oedema, seroma formation and poor wound drainage (Trevor *et al.*, 1992). These problems arise as a consequence of the extensive soft tissue dissection performed at the donor and recipient beds. Passive or active suction drains are placed for at least 3–4 days after surgery to decrease dead space and prevent seroma formation. The application of soft padded bandages protects drains from contamination, decreases dead space and helps to prevent fluid accumulation. Soft padded bandages must be applied without excessive tension to prevent compromise of the flap's pedicle.

Other complications that can occur following the use of an axial pattern flap are distal flap necrosis, dehiscence and infection. Errors in preoperative plan-

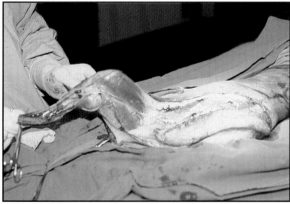

Figure 8.7: This distal tibial wound required a bridging excision over intact skin on the medial side of the femur to connect the donor bed (caudal superficial epigastric flap) to the recipient one.

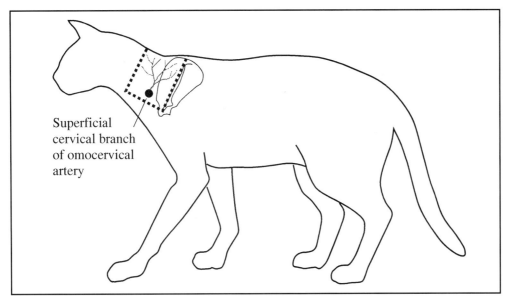

Figure 8.8: The superficial branch of the omocervical artery, used in the omocervical flap originates at the prescapular lymph node and branches craniodorsally. This flap is hardy and very useful in head and neck reconstruction.

ning may lead to a flap that exceeds its vascular territory, resulting in distal necrosis and dehiscence. Postoperative infection is not common, due to the excellent blood supply provided by axial pattern flaps. If infections do occur, dehiscence at the flap-recipient skin edge is an early and prominent clinical feature. Drainage, debridement, lavage and appropriate antibiotic administration are required. With control of local infection, the overall survival of axial pattern skin flaps is not adversely affected.

Head and neck reconstruction

Axial pattern flaps for the reconstruction of head and neck wounds include the omocervical, the superficial temporal and the caudal auricular flaps (Pavletic, 1981; Smith *et al.*, 1991; Fahie and Smith, 1997).

Omocervical flap

The axial pattern flap which is based on the superficial cervical branch of the omocervical artery is often referred to as the omocervical flap. This vessel originates at the prescapular lymph node and radiates craniodorsally (Figure 8.8):

1. After the patient is anesthetized and placed in lateral recumbency with the forelimb, head and neck at natural angles, the cranial shoulder depression is identified (Figure 8.9). This point denotes the emergence of the superficial cervical branch of the omocervical artery from the deep vasculature. A line from the distal aspect of the prescapular lymph node to the acromion defines the ventral flap limit

2. The dorsal edge is formed by the dorsal midline. The cranial limit of the flap is at a point equal to the distance between the cranial shoulder depression and the scapular spine. This border extends dorsally, parallel to the scapular spine. The caudal border is a line parallel with the spine of the scapula. After delineation of the edges with a marker, the flap borders are incised sharply

3. Dissection is commenced at the dorsal border first and the flap is elevated in a dorsal to ventral direction, at a level below the sphincter colli superficialis muscle. As elevation nears the ventral border and the emergence of the superficial cervical artery, dissection must proceed cautiously

4. The donor and recipient beds can be connected by a bridging excision of intact skin lying between these two areas (Figure 8.10a)

5. Following rotation of the flap and drain placement, the flap is tacked into place with a

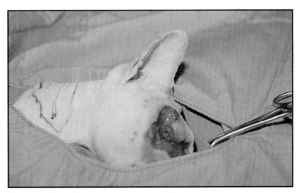

Figure 8.9: This patient required facial reconstruction following extensive orbital and periorbital tumour excision. The cranial shoulder depression is identified as the point of emergence of the superficial branch of the omocervical artery. The flap borders are then delineated. A line from the prescapular lymph node to the acromion defines the ventral flap limit. The dorsal edge is formed by the dorsal midline. The cranial limit of the flap is at a point equal to the distance between the cranial shoulder depression and the scapular spine. This border extends dorsally, parallel to the scapular spine. The caudal border is a line parallel with the scapular spine.

Courtesy of Dr D. Fowler

few simple interrupted sutures, and the remaining edges apposed
6. The donor bed is closed primarily (Figure 8.10b).

This reliable and versatile flap can be used to cover defects that involve the face, head and ear.

For large facial defects, extended omocervical flaps can be raised. This configuration incorporates the contralateral omocervical angiosome, thus creating a flap of sizeable dimensions:

1. Dissection of this extended flap proceeds as in the primary omocervical flap except that the flap borders continue across the dorsal midline to the contralateral shoulder depression
2. At this point, the contralateral superficial branch of the omocervical artery is identified and ligated
3. The flap is then rotated to cover any facial defects that are located rostrally in the nasal, mandibular and maxillary regions.

Superficial temporal flap

An axial pattern flap based on the superficial temporal artery has been described experimentally in cats to reconstruct maxillofacial skin defects (Fahie and Smith, 1997). At the moment, there is minimal clinical information describing the use of this technique. The superficial temporal artery, a terminal branch of the external carotid artery, supplies the frontalis muscle and skin of the temporal area. This vessel emerges at the ventral base of the auricular cartilage and travels dorsally. The lateral orbital rim defines the rostral limit of the flap and the caudal limit is the further caudal aspect of the zygomatic arch. The lateral limits extend to the dorsal orbital rims of the right and left eye. Elevation should be performed below the level of the frontalis muscle. The superficial temporal flap has a similar area of coverage as the omocervical, as both will reach to the rostral nasal area.

Caudal auricular flap

The caudal auricular axial pattern flap, which is based on the sternocleidomastoideus branches of the caudal auricular artery and vein, has been developed in dogs:

1. The sternocleidomastoideus branches originate from the caudal auricular artery at its base on the ventrolateral surface of the annular cartilage. The vessels then course caudally to supply the skin of the neck
2. The sternocleidomastoideus branches can be difficult to identify, and extreme care should be taken when dissecting the base of the flap
3. Harvesting a peninsular axial flap which retains an intact skin border at the base may prevent damage to these fragile vessels. The lateral aspect of the wing of the atlas forms the cranial border of the flap. A line starting at a point

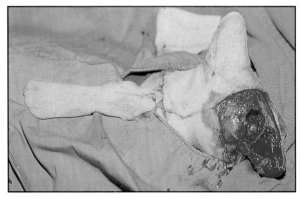
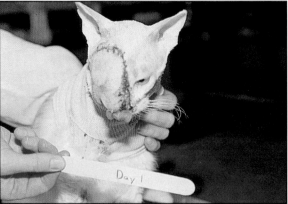

Figure 8.10: *Following elevation and rotation, the flap is sutured into place with a combination of simple interrupted and continuous sutures. The donor bed is closed primarily.*

Courtesy of D. Fowler.

halfway along the scapular spine and extending dorsally defines the caudal border. Two parallel lines extending from the atlas to the scapular spine form the dorsal and ventral limits. Elevation should be performed below the level of the platsyma muscle
4. After rotation, this flap could potentially be used to cover defects of the head and neck.

Forelimb reconstruction

Axial pattern flaps used in the cutaneous reconstruction of forelimb wounds in small animals include the thoracodorsal and superficial brachial flaps (Pavletic, 1981; Shields Henney and Pavletic, 1988; Remedios *et al.*, 1989).

Thoracodorsal flap

The thoracodorsal flap is based on a cutaneous branch of the thoracodorsal artery and vein. These vessels emerge from the intermuscular fascia at the caudal shoulder depression, approximately at the level of the acromion. The vessels then branch and travel caudodorsally (Figure 8.11). The cranial limit of the thoracodorsal flap is defined by a line extending along the scapular spine dorsally. The caudal edge is parallel to the cranial incision and originates at a point approximately equal to the distance from the scapular spine to the caudal shoulder depression. The ventral limit is

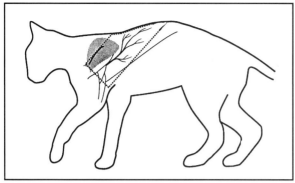

Figure 8.11: The thoracodorsal artery emerges at the caudal shoulder depression and radiates caudodorsally. The cranial limit of the thoracodorsal flap is defined by the scapular spine. The caudal edge is parallel to the cranial incision and originates at a point equal to the distance from the scapular spine to the caudal shoulder depression. The dorsal border is the midline and the ventral border is marked by a line extending from the acromion to the axilla.

marked by a line extending from the acromion caudally to the axilla. The dorsal border is defined by the dorsal midline, although the contralateral angiosome can be harvested to increase flap dimensions:

1. With the patient in lateral recumbency and thoracic limb positioned to simulate a natural standing angle, the borders of the thoracodorsal flap are drawn on the skin surface (Figure 8.12)
2. The location of the vascular pedicle at the caudal shoulder depression should be palpated and identified accordingly
3. Dissection of the thoracodorsal flap starts at the dorsal midline and extends, below the level of the cutaneous trunci muscle, towards the ventral border

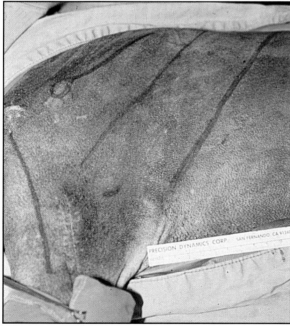

Figure 8.12: The borders of the thoracodorsal flap are drawn on the skin surface with a felt-tipped marker.

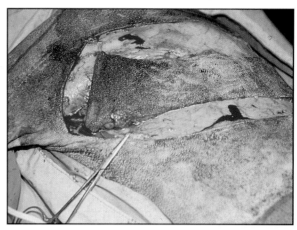

Figure 8.13: The borders of the thoracodorsal flap are incised. Dissection should begin at the dorsal edge and proceed ventrally. At the vascular pedicle (the location is denoted by the haemostat), the surgeon should exercise caution.

4. Initially, surgical elevation of the flap can be rapid, but as the vascular pedicle is approached, cautious and meticulous dissection should be performed (Figure 8.13)
5. To avoid thrombosis and damage, the vascular pedicle does not have to be completely stripped of surrounding fat; rather, isolated only to achieve adequate mobility (Figure 8.14a)
6. After elevation, the thoracodorsal flap is rotated to cover defects of the thorax, shoulder and axillary regions.

However, the most clinically useful application of the thoracodorsal flap is in reconstruction of forelimb defects (Figure 8.14b,c). The rotated thoracodorsal flap reliably covers the mid- to distal antebrachium in dogs and the proximal carpus in cats (Figure 8.15).

Extended thoracodorsal flaps that incorporate adjacent angiosomes have been described. Dissection of these flaps extends over the dorsal midline to the contralateral thoracodorsal vascular pedicle. As the adjacent angiosome depends upon choke communications with the primary flap, distant survival of these extended flaps is less reliable.

Superficial brachial flap

The superficial brachial flap has been described, to reconstruct skin defects involving the lower antebrachium of dogs. The superficial brachial artery emerges at a point 3 cm cranioproximal to the elbow, travels medial to the cephalic vein and branches to the skin of the craniodistal humerus. The base of the flap is centred over the cranial flexor surface of the elbow. The flap extends and tapers proximally to the greater tubercle, parallel to the shaft of the humerus.

The superficial brachial artery is a small diameter vessel and is difficult to identify intraoperatively. These conditions limit the clinical application of this flap as it is susceptible to vascular damage and

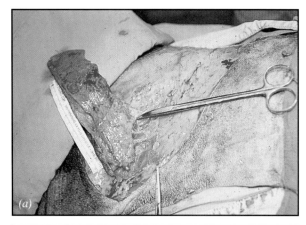

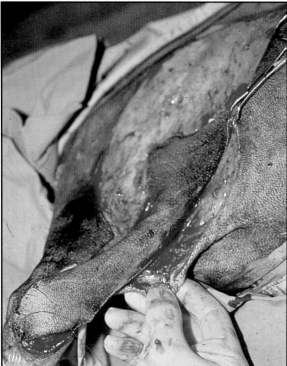

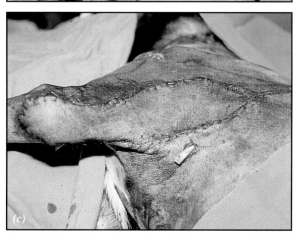

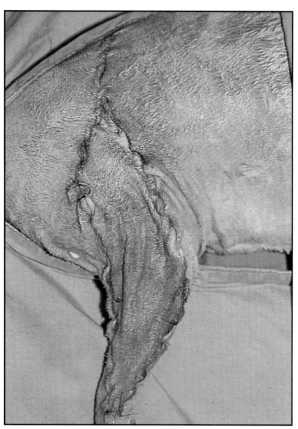

Figure 8.15: *A rotated thoracodorsal flap provides coverage to the proximal carpus in cats.*

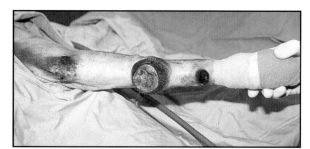

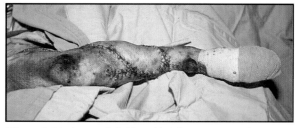

Figure 8.16: *A superficial brachial flap was rotated to cover a wound created following removal of a large tumour involving the caudal aspect of the antebrachium.*

Figure 8.14: *(a) This thoracodorsal flap was harvested in an island configuration to facilitate flap rotation. However, in order to avoid inadvertent injury, the surrounding fat was not stripped from the vascular pedicle. (b) The thoracodorsal flap was then rotated through 180 degrees to cover a decubital ulcer at the point of the elbow. (c) The thoracodorsal flap was sutured in place and a Penrose drain placed to minimize dead space and allow for fluid drainage.*

subsequent necrosis (Figures 8.16 and 8.17). The thoracodorsal flap, which can also be used for forelimb reconstruction, is preferred because of its reliable and robust blood supply.

Should a superficial brachial flap be used, dissection should be performed in the deep subcutaneous layer. Minimal elevation of the flap base should be

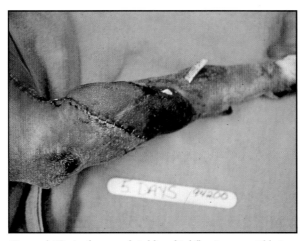

Figure 8.17: As the superficial brachial flap is susceptible to vascular damage, its survival is rather unpredictable. Subsequent flap necrosis has resulted in a large forelimb defect.

undertaken, in an attempt to preserve the superficial brachial vasculature and associated microcirculation. The rotated superficial brachial will cover the foreleg to the distal antebrachium.

Hindlimb reconstruction

Axial pattern flaps that have been described for hindlimb reconstruction in small animals include the caudal superficial epigastric and genicular (Pavletic, 1980; Kostolich and Pavletic, 1987; Remedios *et al.*, 1989).

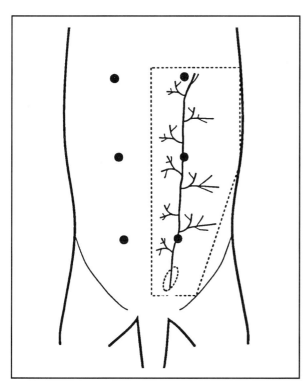

Figure 8.18: The caudal superficial artery emerges at the inguinal ring and supplies the ipsilateral mammary glands, subcutaneous tissue and skin. The caudal flap border is defined by the inguinal ring; the cranial limit is defined by the second mammary gland. The ventral midline is the medial limit and the lateral edge extends from a point twice the distance from the nipple to the ventral midline.

The reverse saphenous conduit flap, which gives off direct cutaneous vessels that supply the hindlimb, is also extremely useful for reconstruction of distal limb wounds (Pavletic *et al.*, 1983).

Caudal superficial epigastric flap

The caudal superficial epigastric is one of the most useful and versatile flaps. The flap is based on the caudal superficial epigastric artery, which is a branch of the external pudendal artery. This vessel emerges at the inguinal ring and courses cranially along the mammary chain, parallel to the ventral midline, to supply the ipsilateral mammary glands, subcutaneous tissue and overlying skin (Figure 8.18). The caudal border of the flap is defined by the inguinal ring. The cranial limit extends to the second mammary gland. The ventral midline delineates the medial limit and the lateral edge extends from a point twice the distance from the nipple to the ventral midline. The flap is created as follows (Figure 8.19):

1. Once the borders of the flap are identified and incised, the caudal superficial epigastric flap is elevated, starting at the cranial border
2. Creation of an island axial pattern flap greatly facilitates transfer of a caudal superficial epigastric flap to a lower limb defect
3. It is essential to undermine the flap just ventral to the aponeurosis of the external abdominal oblique muscle. Once manipulation nears the area of the inguinal ring and location of the vascular pedicle, dissection should proceed with care
4. The donor bed is connected to the recipient area on the limb by a bridging excision of intact skin
5. The flap is then rotated and sutured onto the wound site.

In dogs, depending on the breed conformation, the caudal superficial epigastric flap will cover to mid- or distal tibia. In cats, due to their more pliable skin and their similar body sizes and limb lengths, the caudal superficial epigastic flap can extend to the proximal metatarsus.

Genicular flap

This is described as a peninsular axial pattern flap and is based on the short genicular branch of the saphenous artery and the medial saphenous vein:

- The genicular vessels arise from the saphenous artery, which supplies blood to the medial and lateral skin of the stifle
- The single or paired genicular vessels emerge at the medial aspect of the stifle, running proximolaterally, parallel to the femoral shaft
- The flap is developed from the lateral aspect of the femur. The distal base of the flap extends from just proximal to the patella to immediately

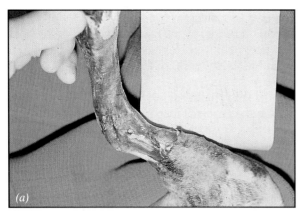
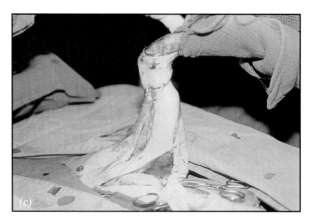
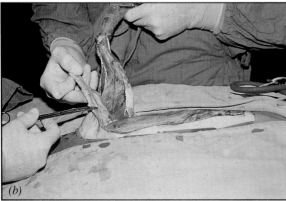
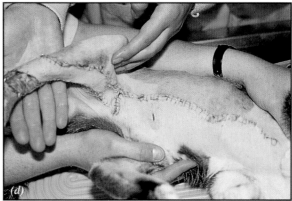

Figure 8.19: *(a) This wound encircles the limb and extends from the distal third of the tibia to mid-metatarsus. (b) The caudal superficial epigastric flap is harvested from the donor bed. A bridging excision is made in the intact skin between the donor bed and the lower limb wound. (c) The caudal superficial epigastric flap is then transferred to the lower limb and sutured in place. (d) At suture removal 14 days following surgery, the entire flap is viable.*

distal to the cranial tibial tuberosity. The cranial and caudal limits run proximally, parallel with the femoral shaft, but taper at the proximal edge as defined by the base of the greater trochanter
- The harvested flap can be rotated to cover defects located on the lateral or medial aspects of the tibia, up to the level of the tibiotarsal joint. The extent of distal cutaneous coverage provided by the genicular flap is comparable with that of the caudal superficial epigastric flap.

Reverse saphenous flap

The reverse saphenous conduit flap has been developed for reconstruction of cutaneous defects involving the tarsus and metatarsus of dogs and cats. This flap is not a true axial pattern flap, but is based on the saphenous vessels, which give off small direct cutaneous vessels that supply the distal limb. Upon development, the blood flow of the flap is reversed through the cranial and caudal branches of the saphenous artery and medial saphenous vein:

1. Preoperatively, measurements are taken to determine the length of flap required to reach and cover the lower limb wound
2. This flap is harvested from the medial aspect of the tibia and is based on direct cutaneous vessels

that supply the flap at the level of the tarsus proximally to the stifle (Figure 8.20)
3. The proximal limit of the flap lies at the level of the patella. A cranial to caudal skin incision is made on the medial aspect of the stifle at this level
4. The saphenous artery and medial saphenous vein are ligated and transected
5. The cranial and caudal limits of the flap are formed by two medial incisions that extend and taper distally to the tibiotarsal joint. These incisions are located approximately 0.5–1 cm cranial and caudal to the borders of the cranial and caudal branches of the saphenous artery and medial saphenous vein
6. This flap is described as a peninsular flap, so the distal skin limit, as defined by the tarsus, is not incised
7. The flap is undermined, starting at the stifle in a distal direction, and extending beneath the saphenous vasculature in the deep subcutaneous layer. To avoid the caudal branch of the saphenous artery and medial saphenous vein, a portion of the medial gastrocnemius muscle may be included in the flap
8. At approximately the distal one-third of the medial tibia, the tibial nerve joins the descending caudal branches of the saphenous artery and

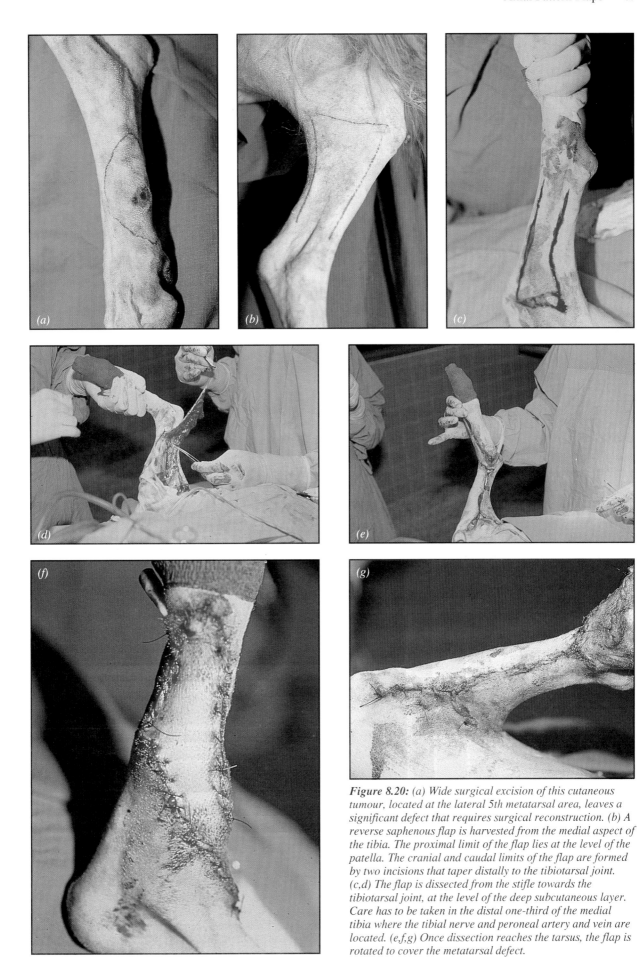

Figure 8.20: *(a) Wide surgical excision of this cutaneous tumour, located at the lateral 5th metatarsal area, leaves a significant defect that requires surgical reconstruction. (b) A reverse saphenous flap is harvested from the medial aspect of the tibia. The proximal limit of the flap lies at the level of the patella. The cranial and caudal limits of the flap are formed by two incisions that taper distally to the tibiotarsal joint. (c,d) The flap is dissected from the stifle towards the tibiotarsal joint, at the level of the deep subcutaneous layer. Care has to be taken in the distal one-third of the medial tibia where the tibial nerve and peroneal artery and vein are located. (e,f,g) Once dissection reaches the tarsus, the flap is rotated to cover the metatarsal defect.*

medial saphenous vein. Dissection should be continued cautiously to avoid nerve injury

9. Frequently, ligation of the peroneal artery and vein are needed to facilitate flap mobility

10. At the level of the tarsus, the flap can be rotated to cover metatarsal defects. Care has to be taken to avoid excessive flap tension at the tibiotarsal joint.

In addition to postoperative complications, such as seroma formation, distal flap necrosis, dehiscence and infection, the reverse saphenous flap is especially susceptible to oedema and congestion. As reversed blood flow is created during flap elevation, venous valvular obstruction and dilatation, and hypertension probably account for both oedema and congestion of the flap (Figure 8.21). It is common for this flap to appear congested for up to 2 weeks after surgery until the formation of venous collateral circulation occurs. The cautious use of soft padded bandages may be beneficial in decreasing oedema.

Perineal reconstruction

Large skin defects involving the perineal area are limited by the lack of available skin and the need to preserve the integrity of the anal and genitourinary areas. Reconstruction can be performed in this area using the caudal superficial epigastric and the deep circumflex iliac flaps (Pavletic, 1981):

1. To reconstruct a perineal defect, elevation of an island caudal superficial epigastric flap is performed as described previously

2. The flap is then rotated 180 degrees to extend coverage to the perineum. Extreme care has to be taken to avoid kinking and minimize tension on the flap pedicle in the highly mobile inguinal region

3. Although a large amount of dead space is created, elimination of this problem through the use of soft padded bandages is difficult in this area. Placement of drains is the best choice to decrease dead space and prevent fluid accumulation in this area

4. Since this region is in close proximity to the highly contaminated anal area, the use of an active closed suction drain is recommended. The drain should exit from a separate stab incision proximal to, and away from, the anus. The suction bulb can be bandaged over the dorsal flank region.

Deep circumflex iliac flap

This is based on the deep circumflex iliac artery, which arises directly from the aorta. The superficial branch of the deep circumflex iliac artery emerges from the lateral abdominal wall, just cranioventral to the iliac wing. Here, it divides into a dorsal and ventral branch. The branches can be used separately for flap development. The dorsal flap is more appropriate for reconstruction of defects located in the flank, lumbar, caudal thorax, lateral thigh and pelvic areas. However, the ventral flap can be harvested as an island flap and used to cover wounds involving the perineal region:

1. To delineate the ventral deep circumflex iliac flap, the animal should be lying in lateral recumbency and the hindlimbs positioned at natural relaxed angles

2. The cranioventral wing of the ilium should be palpated and the borders of the flap are then identified (Figure 8.22). The distal limit is defined by a point midway along the femoral shaft. The dorsal midline forms the dorsal border

3. The caudal incision is formed by a line midway between the cranial edge of the iliac wing and the greater trochanter and directed distally, cranial to the femoral shaft

4. The cranial incision runs parallel with the caudal and is at a point that is equal to the distance between the caudal incision and the cranial iliac wing

5. The flap should be elevated from the deep subcutaneous layer, starting at the distal border

6. Following elevation, the flap can then be rotated and sutured on to the perineal wound. Closed active suction drains are recommended in this location.

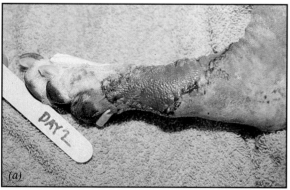
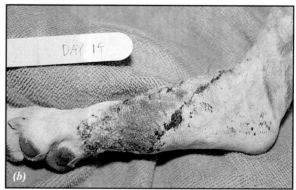

Figure 8.21: (a) Congestion and oedema are common following the rotation of a reverse saphenous flap. Venous valvular obstruction and dilation are probable causes. (b) These problems resolve upon formation of collateral circulation 2–3 weeks after surgery.

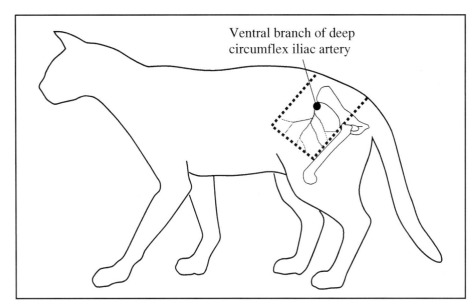

Ventral branch of deep circumflex iliac artery

Figure 8.22: *The ventral deep circumflex iliac flap is used to cover wounds in the perineal region. It is based on the superficial branch of the deep circumflex iliac artery, which emerges at the cranioventral aspect of the ilium. The distal limit is defined by a point midway along the femoral shaft. The dorsal midline forms the dorsal border. The caudal incision is formed by a line midway between the cranial edge of the ilial wing and the greater trochanter. The cranial incision is parallel to the caudal, and is at a point that is equal to the distance between the caudal incision and the cranial iliac wing.*

To cover large perineal defects, an extended ventral deep circumflex iliac flap can be raised by capturing the contralateral angiosome. Dissection of this flap continues over the dorsal midline to the cranioventral border of the ilium where the deep circumflex pedicle originates. This extended flap is used cautiously, as the survival of the distal portion is less predictable than that of the primary flap.

REFERENCES

Fahie MA and Smith MM (1997) Axial pattern flap based on the superficial temporal artery in cats: an experimental study. *Veterinary Surgery* **26**, 86-89

Kostolich M and Pavletic MM (1987) Axial pattern flap based on the genicular branch of the saphenous artery in the dog. *Veterinary Surgery* **16**, 217-222

Madison JB, Donawick WJ, Johnston DE and Orsini RA (1989) The use of skin expansion to repair cosmetic defects in animals. *Veterinary Surgery* **18**, 15-21

Pavletic MM (1980) Caudal superficial epigastric arterial pedicle grafts in the dog. *Veterinary Surgery* **9**, 103-107

Pavletic MM (1981) Canine axial pattern flaps, using the omocervical, thoracodorsal and deep circumflex iliac direct cutaneous arteries. *American Journal of Veterinary Research* **42**, 391-406

Pavletic MM, Watters J, Henry RW and Nafe LA (1983) Reverse saphenous conduit flap in the dog. *Journal of the American Veterinary Medical Association* **182**, 380-389

Remedios AM, Bauer MS and Bowen CV (1989) Thoracodorsal and caudal superficial epigastric axial pattern skin flaps in cats. *Veterinary Surgery* **18**, 380-385

Shields Henney LH and Pavletic MM (1988) Axial pattern flaps based on the superficial brachial artery in the dog. *Veterinary Surgery* **17**, 311-317

Smith MM, Payne JT, Moon ML and Freeman LE (1991) Axial pattern flap based on the caudal auricular artery in dogs. *American Journal of Veterinary Research* **52**, 922-925

Taylor GI and Palmer JH (1987) The vascular territories (angiosomes) of the body: experimental study and clinical applications. *British Journal of Plastic Surgery* **67**, 177-187

Trevor PB, Smith MM, Waldron DR and Hedlund CS (1992) Clinical evaluation of axial pattern skin flaps in dogs and cats: 19 cases (1981-1990). *Journal of the American Veterinary Medical Association* **210**, 608-612

CHAPTER NINE

Skin Grafting

Richard A.S. White

INDICATIONS

The use of free skin grafts is confined primarily to the reconstruction of large skin deficits involving the extremities of the limbs, which present the surgeon with some unique problems. Elsewhere in the body, the primary solution for dealing with skin deficits is simple coaption of the wound but this is usually precluded for limb sites due to the lack of adjacent mobile skin. Secondary healing can be allowed to proceed for some limb skin defects, although there is a risk of developing unsightly scars and those in the vicinity of joints may seriously impair limb function should excessive scar tissue form. Other options include local or random flaps which may be indicated for the reconstruction of some larger wounds but their use is again restricted in the case of limbs by the limited availability of adjacent skin. Heterotopic pedicle grafts, using microvascular anastomosis to relocate axial flaps based on a single arteriovenous supply, can provide an alternative solution but are used infrequently because of the complexity of the surgical procedure (see Chapter 11). Direct flaps offer an alternative solution in some cases by positioning the limb deficit under pedicles of skin created on the flank, although this may not be appropriate for the temperament of all patients.

In many cases therefore, free skin grafts provide the only viable alternative to the problem of reconstructing some of the larger skin deficits involving the distal limb. It should always be borne in mind, however, before undertaking a skin graft, that the technique can be very time-consuming, not only in terms of the surgery but also in the postoperative care. Since the successful outcome of the graft can never be guaranteed, it pays to consider carefully all other possible alternatives before selecting a skin graft.

TYPES OF SKIN GRAFT

Skin grafts are classified in two ways. First, according to the depth of skin harvested (Figure 9.1) as:

- Full thickness (containing the epidermis and the entire dermis) or
- Split thickness (containing the epidermis and only part of the dermis).

Full thickness grafts

Full thickness skin grafts are generally considered to be the more suitable depth of graft for small animal reconstructive use. They are robust and capable of withstanding considerable handling during collection and positioning over the recipient site. Because the grafts retain all the dermal structures they can provide far more cosmetic skin regrowth in the longer term. Their greater tissue content, however, means that the nutritional requirements during the 'take' period (see below) are considerably more fastidious than those of the thinner split thickness graft and hence they 'take' less readily.

Split thickness grafts

Split thickness skin grafts contain the epidermis and part of the dermis. They are sometimes referred to as Thiersch grafts and can be further subclassified as thin, medium or thick split thickness depending on the depth of dermis harvested in the graft. Despite their widespread use in human plastic reconstructions, split thickness grafts have a number of important disadvantages in small animal surgery and are used infrequently. They are rather fragile by comparison with full thickness grafts and require considerably more care during collection and placement. Due to the variable absence of the dermal structures the grafted sites tend to have poor durability, a greater tendency to contracture and to produce sparse hair regrowth. Equally important, the donor site heals by epithelialization and hence its final cosmetic appearance is poor. Although they are potentially useful for the reconstruction of very large wounds where the supply of donor skin is at a premium, it is unusual to be unable to harvest sufficient skin to permit full thickness grafting in the majority of cases. The complexity of accurate collection and the significant cost of the harvesting equipment tend to argue additionally against the use of split thickness grafts in small animals.

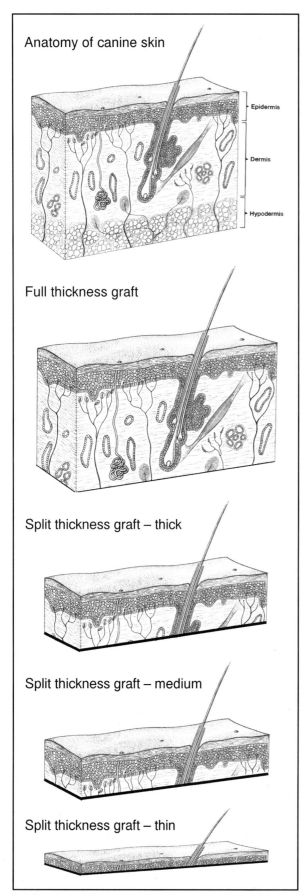

Anatomy of canine skin

Full thickness graft

Split thickness graft – thick

Split thickness graft – medium

Split thickness graft – thin

Figure 9.1: *Types of skin graft. Classification according to skin depth.*

Copyright © R.A.S. White.

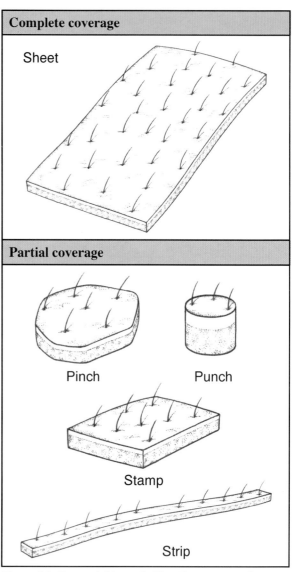

Complete coverage

Sheet

Partial coverage

Pinch   Punch

Stamp

Strip

Figure 9.2: *Types of skin graft. Classification according to wound coverage.*

Copyright © R.A.S. White.

Secondly, skin grafts are classified according to the extent of wound coverage they offer (Figure 9.2) and the manner in which they are prepared as:

- Sheet grafts, providing full wound coverage, or
- Pinch, punch, stamp or strip grafts, for partial coverage of granulating wounds.

Sheet grafts
Sheet grafts are the most frequently used skin grafts in small animal reconstruction. They provide complete coverage of the wound and will ultimately provide the most functional and cosmetically acceptable result.

Pinch, punch, stamp and strip grafts
These provide partial coverage of granulating wounds. They are used simply as a means of promoting healing of granulation tissue by vastly increasing the surface of epithelializing tissue within the wound.

Their collection and placement is labour intensive and they provide a poor final cosmetic and functional result in a wound that heals largely by epithelialization and contraction.

HARVESTING THE GRAFT

Ideal donor sites for skin grafts in the small animal species should have:

- Durable skin of a suitable thickness (usually avoiding the thin skin over the ventral abdomen)
- An abundant supply of easily mobilized skin, to allow easy and cosmetic closure of the donor site
- Hair of a colour, length and density similar to that which it is intended to replace at the recipient site (less important for split thickness grafts).

The flank usually satisfies most of these criteria and offers the best opportunity to remove a sufficiently large area of skin to cover wounds involving the limb. In the case of full thickness grafts, however, hair length from this site can be noticeably greater than that which it replaces. The skin should be collected under strictly aseptic conditions and, once harvested, should be rolled in saline- or antibiotic-soaked sponges to prevent desiccation until required. Harvested skin prepared in this fashion can be preserved for several days by refrigeration at 4°C .

Full thickness grafts
Full thickness grafts are collected by elevating the skin, including its hypodermal attachments, from the loose fatty tissue below, without disturbing the underlying panniculus muscles. This can be more easily accomplished with the use of skin hooks or fine monofilament nylon stay sutures strategically placed at the periphery of the graft as it is elevated. The need to pre-cut the graft in the shape of the recipient wound will depend on whether the graft is to be subsequently meshed or not. Meshing enables the sheet to be manipulated to the outline of the recipient bed and requires minimal pre-shaping whereas unmeshed sheet grafts are less flexible and require accurate pre-shaping. However, even unmeshed sheets have some degree of elasticity which will permit stretching to accommodate small irregularities. Where a graft is to be pre-shaped to a template it is best achieved with the help of a moist surgical swab cut to the outline of the recipient area and then laid over the donor skin. The general outline of the graft to be harvested is marked with a sterile marker, allowing some overlap (0.5–1.0 cm) to ensure collection of an adequate area. Donor sites require primary surgical repair with closure of the subcutaneous tissues.

Occasionally there may be an indication for the use of pinch, punch, stamp or strip grafts although, as already indicated, they provide a very poor cosmetic result and are limited to partial coverage of granulating wounds. These are normally harvested in full thickness. Pinch grafts are harvested by scalpel excision of small areas of skin raised by means of hypodermic needle. Punch grafts are most easily collected by means of the Keyes biopsy punch. Stamps are removed as small rectangular sheets, whilst strips are collected as 0.5 cm wide lengths.

Split thickness grafts
Split thickness grafts dictate accurate collection through the dermal layer itself by means of a blade pre-set to the required depth. A wide array of instruments are available for this, including the Humbly and Silva knives and also the Brown dermatome (Figure 9.3); the former are hand-held whilst dermatomes are either pneumatically or electrically driven. Most instruments have some device for pre-setting the depth of cut and, with the skin held in tension, the blade is either drawn to and fro across the surface or progresses by means of an oscillating blade. Split thickness grafts are quite fragile and should be carefully supported on a moist dressing until positioned over the recipient site.

PREPARING THE GRAFT

Once harvested, the underlying hypodermal and loose adipose tissue is carefully removed from the full thickness graft with fine scissors until the pigment of the dermal layer is apparent, in order to maximize subsequent vascular access to the graft from the recipient bed. Less ideally, this can be performed by careful scraping with a scalpel blade but overly vigorous scarification of the dermal structures should be avoided. The graft can be laid on the bevelled surface of a skin

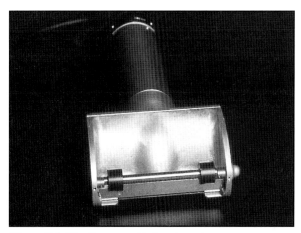

Figure 9.3: *The Brown oscillating dermatome.*

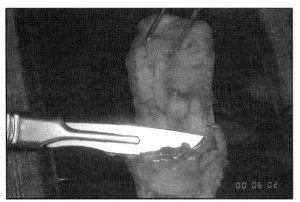

Figure 9.4: *Removal of hypodermal tissue. A skin graft board with the unwanted tissue being removed by scalpel.*

Copyright © R.A.S. White.

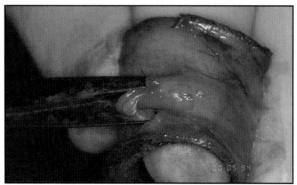

Figure 9.5: *Removal of hypodermal tissue. The graft is draped over the surgeon's finger to permit removal of the unwanted tissue by careful trimming with scissors.*

Copyright © R.A.S. White.

graft board (Figure 9.4) to achieve this, although many surgeons prefer to drape the graft over their fingers whilst the tissue is removed (Figure 9.5). Sheet grafts can now be further prepared as unmeshed, meshed or 'pie-crusted' (Figure 9.6).

Unmeshed sheets

Unmeshed sheets are left intact after removal of the hypodermal tissues so that there is no disruption to contiguity of the dermal sheet. This type of graft provides potentially for the best cosmetic result and in the event that there is full 'take' there will be little to distinguish the grafted area from normal skin elsewhere. Despite this apparent advantage, there are some significant drawbacks which make unmeshed grafts a rather impractical and infrequently used option. The most important of these is that the intact sheet provides no route for the drainage of the exudate which inevitably accumulates between it and the recipient site during the 'take' period. This fluid promotes lifting of the graft from the recipient bed and may lead to its eventual loss. This can be countered by aspirating exudate from under the graft using a hypodermic needle on a daily basis or by the use of a fine suction drain placed under the graft (see Chapter 6), but these options are likely to be less successful than a system of free drainage through the graft itself. Less importantly, unmeshed grafts must be pre-cut to the outline of the recipient site since they have only limited ability to stretch to wound shapes.

Meshed sheets

Meshed sheets are prepared by the creation of perforations through the entire thickness of the skin. This can be performed by hand or mechanically by means of a meshing table (Figure 9.7) or roller mesher. Meshing can be complete, partial or 'pie-crusted' and confers a number of significant advantages on the graft:

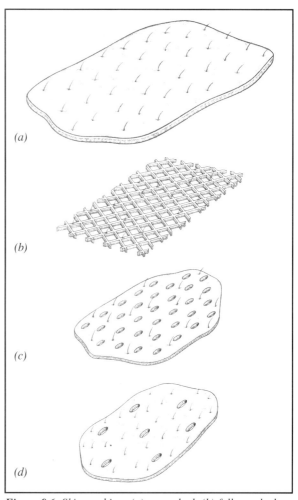

Figure 9.6: *Skin meshing: (a) unmeshed; (b) fully meshed; (c) partially meshed; (d) 'pie-crusted'.*

Copyright © R.A.S. White.

*   The graft has much greater flexibility and elasticity which enables it to be easily shaped to the outline of irregular wounds. In the wider regions of the wound the meshings of graft can

be fully 'opened' to cover the required area whilst in the narrower regions the meshes are left 'unopened'. This obviates the need to pre-shape the graft and most wound shapes can be accommodated from a simple rectangle whose general dimensions approximate those of the recipient bed

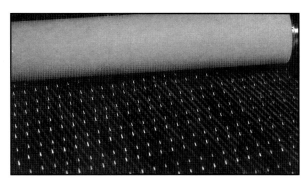

Figure 9.7: *A table meshing instrument. The graft is laid over the table which consists of parallel rows of blades and then firmly rolled with the Teflon® rolling pin to produce a fully meshed graft.*

Copyright © R.A.S. White.

- The greater flexibility of the graft also enables it to conform closely to uneven wound surfaces. Meshed grafts will readily conform to wounds with convex surfaces (e.g. over the elbow, hock) without the need for copious additional sutures through the graft surface to ensure immobilization
- The graft can be expanded simply by pulling the meshing open, allowing it to cover a greater area of wound. Meshing may therefore help to solve the problem of covering large wounds in situations where the amount of skin available for grafting is limited
- By far the greatest advantage of meshing lies in its inherent capacity to permit ongoing drainage of any exudate from the recipient surface during the 'take' phase. The greater the number of mesh openings and the wider they are opened, the greater is the potential for this fluid to drain without interfering with 'take'. However, the areas of the wound under the mesh openings do not have any dermal covering and hence these regions heal secondarily by granulation, contraction and epithelialization, the consequence of which is an area of alopecia. The goal is therefore to achieve a balance between providing adequate drainage and accomplishing a good cosmetic result.

'Pie-crusted sheets'
'Pie-crusted' sheets represent a compromise between meshing (which provides drainage) and leaving the graft as an intact sheet (for optimal cosmetic results). 'Pie-crusting' describes the preparation of the graft by making a limited number of stab incisions through the graft, sufficient to permit adequate drainage whilst causing minimal damage to the cosmetic result.

Pinch, punch, stamp and strip grafts
Pinch, punch, stamp and strip grafts should also have the hypodermal tissue removed, as for sheet grafts, although this is often difficult and time consuming due to their small size and multiplicity. Drainage of

exudate from the wound is not a consideration for these grafts since the wound surface itself remains largely open.

THE RECIPIENT SITE

A major determinant in the success of free skin grafting is the proper preparation of the recipient site. Sites should be well supplied with the active capillary vessels necessary to provide nutritional support and ultimately revascularization of the graft. All non-viable tissue debris or epithelialized tissue which may prevent capillary ingress into the graft should be removed. Any major bacterial contamination likely to lead to infection should be dealt with prior to grafting. Suitable recipient tissues for skin grafting may be: healthy granulation tissue; surgically clean wounds; or fresh surgical wounds.

Granulation tissue
Granulation tissue is an ideal graft recipient tissue, since it contains an abundant supply of vascular capillaries in a stable matrix of collagen ready to support the overlying graft. Its appearance in the wound within 3–6 days of the original injury is an indication that all septic processes have been controlled and that grafting can proceed safely. Although grafting can be considered as soon as granulation tissue first appears in the wound it is often delayed for several days until the wound is completely covered and the prospects for successful 'take' are considerably increased. Chronic granulation tissue that remains ungrafted, on the other hand, is less likely to support a graft because its capillary content is significantly reduced by the increasing proportion of connective tissue. This can, however, readily be converted to healthy tissue with a well vascularized surface by surgical debridement immediately prior to grafting or better still, 24 hours before grafting to minimize the risk of haematoma or seroma development. Where the granulation tissue is less chronically inactive, simple mechanical debridement for 1–2 days prior to grafting will be sufficient to promote surface revascularization (Figures 9.8 and 9.9). All vascular oozing should be controlled using diathermy to minimize the risk of fluid accumulating below the graft.

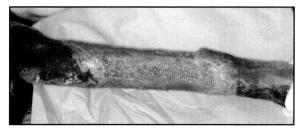

Figure 9.8: *Preparation of granulation tissue for grafting. This degloving injury is covered with chronic granulation and will not support a skin graft.*

Copyright © R.A.S. White.

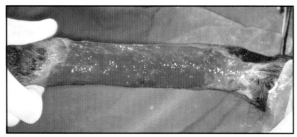

Figure 9.9: *Preparation of granulation tissue for grafting. The same wound as that in Figure 9.8 following wet-to-dry dressing over a 48-hour period. The granulation tissue now appears much more active and is suitable for grafting.*

Copyright © R.A.S. White.

Surgically 'clean' wounds

Recent wounds that have been debrided and retain a suitable vascular supply can undergo immediate grafting. Examples of this include degloving and avulsion wounds in which the skin has been removed but is still available to be replaced in its original location. Contamination of the wound and the subsequent collection of exudate are, however, considerably greater risks in this type of recipient bed.

Fresh surgical wounds

Fresh surgical wounds are frequently overlooked as potential sites for skin grafting. They are very suitable recipient sites providing that the wound is well vascularized (Figure 9.10). The development of haematomas or serous exudate below the graft is, however, a much more frequent problem and it is essential that some kind of provision is made for drainage. Delaying the graft by even as little as 24–48 hours after the original surgery to encourage early granulation substantially reduces this problem.

APPLICATION OF THE GRAFT

Unmeshed or 'pie-crusted' sheets

Unmeshed or 'pie-crusted' sheets require pre-shaping to the recipient site (Figure 9.11) allowing a few millimetres overlap on all edges to provide for any contracture as the graft 'takes'. Grafts are sutured in place with loosely applied and widely spaced simple interrupted 2 metric (3/0) monofilament nylon around their periphery. Anchoring the graft so that it is under a little tension ensures good contact with the recipient surface but care should be taken to avoid over-tensioning. In the case of large or convex wounds it is also wise to place loose mattress sutures through the graft itself into the underlying granulation tissue or wound to prevent graft movement. A fine suction drain should be implanted to prevent the fluid accumulation in the case of unmeshed sheets.

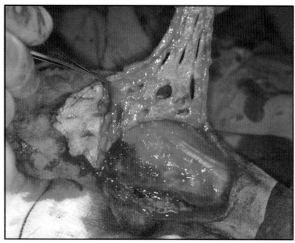

Figure 9.10: *Fresh surgical wounds can be grafted immediately, although the problems of seroma development are likely to be more severe. A partially meshed graft is placed over a wound created by the resection of a benign tumour over a carpus following careful haemostasis.*

Copyright © R.A.S. White.

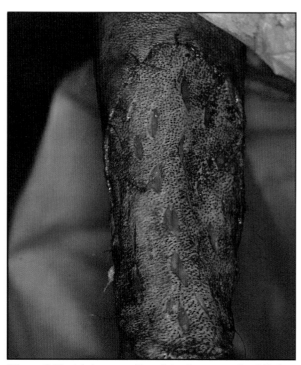

Figure 9.11: *A 'pie-crusted' graft in situ over a distal limb deficit. Note that some sutures are placed through the graft itself to the recipient bed to ensure stability.*

Copyright © R.A.S. White.

Meshed sheets

Meshed sheets do not require pre-shaping and the graft can be placed over the wound and expanded to fit the wound as necessary with the edges left overlapping the wound (Figure 9.12). The maximal expansion of the meshed graft is usually up to 2–4 times the original width of the graft but this is achieved at the expense of some reduction in graft length. Grafts are anchored as for other sheet grafts.

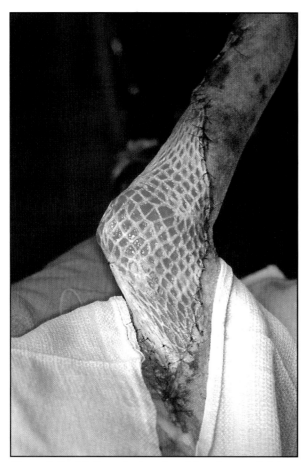

Figure 9.12: A fully meshed graft positioned over a deficit over the elbow. The graft has been expanded to provide wound coverage. Note how in the fully meshed form the graft conforms to the convex wound surface.

Partial coverage grafts

Although stamps and strips can be sutured in place, pinch and punch grafts cannot be attached to wound surfaces in the manner described above and can only be positioned by firmly embedding them in granulation tissue. Punch grafts are placed in holes cut in the granulation tissue with a biopsy punch; pinch grafts are wedged into stab holes; stamps are positioned in square holes; whilst strips are placed in longitudinal grooves. All partial coverage grafts are inherently unstable and require careful pressure bandaging until they gain stability at the end of 24–48 hours.

GRAFT 'TAKE'

The processes whereby a graft survives from the time that it is placed over the recipient site until it becomes fully revascularized by the underlying capillaries are often collectively termed graft 'take'. They involve much more than simple ingrowth of new capillaries from the recipient bed. Two separate, but interrelated, processes are important for the take of a graft: adherence and nutrition.

Adherence

Adherence refers to the development of a 'scaffold' of fibrin between the graft and the underlying recipient surface. The fibrin is exuded from the recipient surface within a few hours of the graft covering it and serves not only to anchor the graft but also provides a means of support for the subsequent ingrowth of new capillaries from the recipient tissue. The fibrin is progressively replaced by fibrous tissue, further adding to the stability of the grafted skin during the first week. The process of fibrin adherence is essential for the subsequent processes which contribute to graft nutrition.

Nutrition

Nutrition of the graft comprises three separate processes:

- Plasmatic imbibition
- Inosculation
- Revascularization.

Plasmatic imbibition

Plasmatic imbibition, sometimes called plasmatic circulation, occurs during the first 2–3 days. The graft behaves rather like physiological blotting paper at this stage and absorbs the fibrinogen-free serum proteins and erythrocytes which are exuded from the recipient surface. As a result it takes on an oedematous appearance and is often darkly pigmented through absorption of haem degradation products. The swelling of the graft at this stage can be sufficient to cause the mesh openings in partially meshed and 'pie-crusted' grafts to close over, thereby impeding the drainage of any exudate. The rather unhealthy appearance of the graft at this stage is often mistaken for early rejection. Plasmatic imbibition, however, is thought to be important in providing early nutritional support until capillary ingrowth begins to develop.

Inosculation

Inosculation is the development of a rudimentary vascular circulation within the graft and begins around the second or third day. New capillary buds develop from the recipient tissue and cross the fibrin scaffold into the graft. Instead of simply distributing throughout the tissue they are able to locate the old vessels in the graft and anastomose with these. This process of connection between the new capillaries and old blood vessels is thought to provide sluggish and disorganized movement of blood. It is not clear how important this process is in contributing to the long-term survival of the graft but it may be responsible for the more viable appearance that successful grafts take on towards the middle of the first week. It is vitally important that the graft remains immobilized during this period to enable this delicate vascular 're-plumbing' to take place.

Revascularization

Revascularization, or vascular penetration, may take a further 1–2 weeks to complete, by which time the healthy appearance of the graft underlines the re-establishment of circulation in the skin.

CARE OF THE GRAFT

It is comparatively easy to prepare the recipient bed, harvest the graft and position it over the recipient bed. However, it is considerably more difficult to ensure that what happens over the following few days results in a successful 'take'. The survival of a skin graft depends on optimization of the conditions that promote adherence and nutrition and it is essential that the surgeon fully appreciates all of the stages involved in graft growth described above in order to achieve this.

Dressing and bandaging

Suitable dressing and bandaging during the period of graft 'take' is critical and serves a number of functions:

- Promotes good contact between graft and recipient tissue
- Minimizes graft movement
- Removes exudate from the region of the graft
- Prevents soiling and bacterial contamination of the wound.

The use of 'tie over', or bolus, dressings (see Chapter 5) has been advocated to create firm uniform downward pressure across grafts but these are difficult to attach to circumferential limb wounds. Instead, a properly constructed bandage support should be used comprising:

- *A low-adherent contact layer*, usually consisting of a commercially available perforated silicon sheet (Figure 9.13) or a plastic sheet backed with an absorbent material which allows the dressing to be removed regularly with minimal disruption of the graft during dressing changes
- *An absorbent intermediate layer* (e.g. cotton wool) to remove any exudate from the wound and to provide support to limit movement of the limb
- *An outer protective layer* into which can be incorporated a gutter splint for additional immobilization of the limb during the first 5 days (Figure 9.14).

Graft inspection

It is essential to prevent exudate from accumulating below the graft by regular dressing changes, since excess exudate will not only mechanically interfere with 'take' but also provide an excellent medium for bacterial proliferation. The first dressing change is normally undertaken within 48 hours of grafting and, since graft adherence is only partially developed at this time, great care should be taken to avoid disturbing the graft as the contact layer is peeled away (Figure 9.15). The frequency of subsequent changes will depend on the amount of exudate produced by the graft site but normally changes every 24–48 hours are appropriate during the first week. Fresh surgical wounds are more productive and will certainly require daily changes during this period.

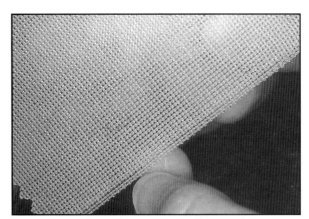

Figure 9.13: *A low-adherence contact layer, in this case a silicon mesh dressing, is placed over the graft before bandaging.*

Copyright © R.A.S. White.

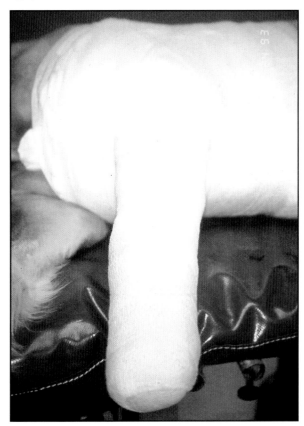

Figure 9.14: *The graft site on the limb is placed within a well padded Robert Jones bandage to prevent movement at the graft site.*

Copyright © R.A.S. White.

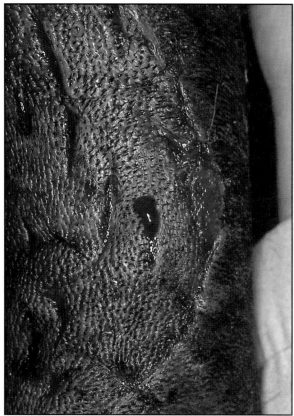

Figure 9.15: A full thickness graft 48 hours after placement. Note the oedematous appearance of the graft due to serum imbibition which is now causing the mesh openings to close. Fluid from the recipient bed can be seen exuding through the mesh openings. The dark red/bluish colour is normal at this stage.

Copyright © R.A.S. White.

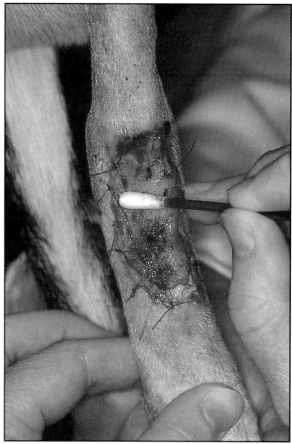

Figure 9.16: During the first 5–7 days coagulated debris should be carefully removed from the mesh openings and accumulated exudate removed by rolling a cotton bud along the graft.

Copyright © R.A.S. White.

At each dressing change the graft should be inspected for any indication of fluid accumulating between it and the wound. This is most likely to be a problem in the case of unmeshed and 'pie-crusted' sheets, and early detection and intervention is important to save a graft before it becomes completely separated from the wound. In the case of unmeshed grafts, exudate can be removed by careful aspiration using a fine hypodermic needle if a fine suction drain has not been placed. For meshed and pie-crusted grafts, a cotton bud should be used to open carefully each mesh which may have become plugged with coagulated exudate; by carefully rolling the bud along the graft with light downward pressure, any accumulated fluid can be expressed through the mesh openings (Figure 9.16).

Longer-term care

Although graft 'take' will normally be obvious within the first 4–5 days, ongoing care of the graft will be necessary for several weeks. Once the graft is firmly in place the need for immobilization declines and dressings can normally be progressively reduced in frequency and quantity depending on the graft appearance. A low-adherence contact layer and absorbent second layer should be maintained until all exudation has ceased. In some grafts there may be accumulation of dried debris on the surface of the graft which can be managed by *very careful* wet-to-dry dressing for 24–48 hours. It should be remembered that grafted skin is not fully functional, nor is it resistant to normal abrasive use for 4–6 weeks. It should be treated with care during this period to minimize the development of excessive connective tissue within the graft which will limit its cosmetic and functional result. Grafts are often lacking in natural secretions during their early life and frequent application of lanolin-based creams will improve its appearance and functionality. Patients often find the graft site pruritic during its first few weeks and steps should be taken to prevent late graft loss through self-trauma.

COMPLICATIONS

The most common causes of graft failure include: an inadequately vascularized recipient bed; movement; and infection. Where graft loss does occur, it is not usually apparent for the first 3–4 days post grafting. Initially, as the graft fails it will become blanched but then quickly progress to a black, dehydrated appearance

(Figure 9.17) unless remedial action is taken. Once the limit of the graft necrosis can be definitively identified, the dead tissue should be trimmed away as soon as possible to minimize the risk of bacterial proliferation and prevent loss of any remaining graft.

Fluid accumulating below the graft normally has a serosanguinous appearance and although it demands rapid removal if the graft is to be saved it does not necessarily indicate imminent loss provided that there is no indication of purulent content.

Some grafts appear to discard their epidermal layer after 5-7 days and an apparently complete graft will seem to separate from the recipient bed, leaving no obvious evidence of 'take' in the wound. This can be disconcerting but usually a 'ghost' outline of the dermal graft will appear within the next week and the graft progress on to a completely satisfactory result.

Infection

Infection associated with skin grafting is uncommon if aseptic techniques are properly observed. Where infection does occur, *Pseudomonas* or *Klebsiella* organisms are often implicated and can lead to rapid and disastrous graft loss. The septic process may result in sufficient exudation from the wound to separate it physically from the graft whilst at the same time activating the fibrinolytic system which dissolves the all-important fibrin attachment between recipient bed and graft. Selective resection may salvage any unaffected regions but often the process is rapid and comprehensive.

The incidence of sepsis can be minimized by attention to aseptic technique at both donor and recipient sites. Pre-soaking the graft in antibiotic solutions is reported to reduce the incidence of sepsis although the use of systemic antibiotics is probably more rational. Topical antibiotics can be used if the risk of infection is perceived to be significant; these are best delivered by spray and should be active against Pseudomonads and β-lactamase-producing organisms (see also Chapter 5).

Figure 9.18 describes some methods of 'trouble shooting' for graft problems.

INTERPRETING GRAFT APPEARANCE

During the period of 'take' the graft will undergo a variety of physical changes which can be difficult to interpret and occasionally lead to viable grafts being discarded prematurely.

What to expect

- From Day 1 onwards the graft should be surprisingly well fixed to the recipient bed and capable of withstanding reasonable disturbance during dressing changes
- During the first 2-3 days as plasmatic imbibition peaks, the graft will become engorged and oedematous, its colour will darken and regions of the graft will take on a range of hues from light through dark blue. At this stage, areas of blue coloration are healthy and the surgeon should not be tempted to discard!
- Towards the end of the first week the graft will become less oedematous and assume a pinker appearance as modest circulation begins; however, it will be several days before it has a well vascularized appearance
- Signs of hair regrowth will normally appear towards the end of the second or third week, although this is variable and complete regrowth may take several weeks.

What not to expect

- Any movement of the graft evident during dressing changes is a concerning feature, although it is perhaps less disastrous during the first 24-48 hours, whilst there is still potential for plasmatic imbibition to continue to

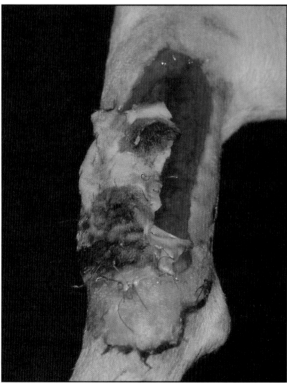

Figure 9.17: An entire full thickness graft showing failure at 5 days post grafting. Note the blanched white and black areas indicative of necrosis. Failure in this case was due to inadequate preparation of an underlying indolent granulation tissue in a burn wound.

Problem and cause	Pathophysiology	Management
Fluid accumulation below the graft All recipient beds exude some fluid but excessive fluid may be produced after: - poor haemostasis in the wound surface - grafting over fresh wounds	Fluid separates the graft from the recipient bed and removes the serum nutritional source The fibrin scaffold is broken down and new capillary growth is prevented	Drainage can be achieved by: - using a meshed graft - placing an active suction drain below the graft - aspirating fluid with a hypodermic needle on a daily basis
Graft movement Inadequate immobilization of the graft: - poor suture placement - insufficient bandaging to prevent limb movement	Some minor movement of the graft within the first 24 hours is acceptable and does not necessarily indicate graft loss Subsequent movement will lead to shearing of new capillaries growing into the graft and failure of revascularization	The graft should be sutured under slight tension with mattress sutures through the graft to the recipient surface if necessary An appropriate three-layer Robert Jones bandage should be employed during the first week
Infection Poor aseptic technique Pre-existing infection in the graft bed	Toxin release and cell death causes lysis of the fibrin scaffold and failure of revascularization	Good aseptic technique Pre-soaking graft in antibiotic solution Systemic antibiotic therapy Rapid resection of any areas of infection
Graft necrosis *Early* Inadequate debridement of the dermal side of the graft Poorly vascularized recipient bed (e.g. indolent granulation tissue) *Late* Graft dressings overly tight Impaired systemic health of the patient	Early failure (first 3–4 days) through poor nutrition is due to impaired serum exudation/imbibition. Later failure (beyond 3–4 days) indicates failure of revascularization	Check dressings Resect non-viable areas as soon as apparent Start over if the cause is a poor granulation bed

Figure 9.18: Trouble shooting for skin grafting.

support the graft without total stability and for re-establishment of adherence
- Beyond this period, any instability in the graft will result in the failure of angiogenesis
- Blue coloration is an encouraging feature of graft 'take' but other colours, notably blanched white or black, usually indicate graft death
- Some grafts may show signs of superficial infection but any evidence of any purulent fluid under the graft is usually a disastrous development and graft salvage proves impossible in most cases.

THE COSMETIC RESULT

The final cosmetic appearance of grafted skin in small animals depends primarily on the amount of dermal tissue applied and which 'takes' at the graft site. This determines not only the density of hair follicles grafted but also the other dermal structures which contribute to

the long-term strength and durability of the graft. In the first instance, therefore, the dermal component is determined by the depth of skin harvested for the graft:

- Full thickness grafts contain their full complement of hair follicles and hence have the potential for complete regrowth, although even these can be significantly reduced in number by over-enthusiastic removal of hypodermal and dermal tissue during preparation
- Split thickness grafts retain fewer hair follicles and can never provide complete hair regrowth.

Dermal density is also determined by the proportion of the wound which heals by epithelialization, since these regions will contain no hair follicles and detract from the cosmetic result:

- Fully meshed sheets with wide open meshes heal with a significant proportion of epithelialized skin and hence have a sparse hair covering (Figure 9.19)

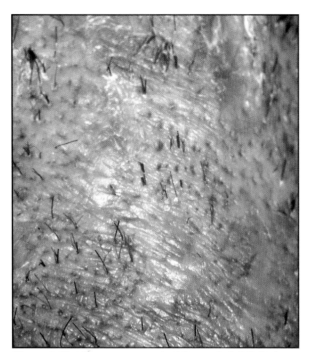

Figure 9.19: The appearance of a fully meshed, full thickness graft at 21 days. The areas of early hair regrowth are interspersed with regions of epithelialization corresponding to the mesh openings. Widely opened, fully meshed grafts result in sparse hair growth.

Copyright © R.A.S. White.

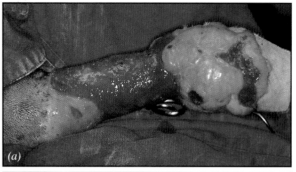

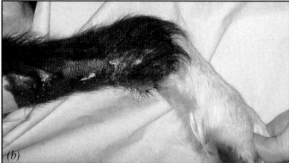

Figure 9.20: (a) A degloving injury overlying the distal limb. Carpal function is limited by exuberant scar tissue. (b) Two months after grafting with a full thickness 'pie-crusted' graft. Hair regrowth is good and carpal function restored. 'Pie-crusted' meshing achieves near-normal final hair density.

Copyright © R.A.S. White.

- 'Pie-crusted' sheets result in almost normal hair regrowth (Figure 9.20)
- Unmeshed skin provides the densest result in theory
- Partial coverage techniques produce the most inferior results of all, with most of the wound healing by epithelialization.

FURTHER READING

Pavletic MM (1992) Free grafts. In *Atlas of Reconstructive Surgery*, ed. MM Pavletic, pp.241–261. Lippincott, Philadelphia

Swaim SF (1993) Skin grafting. In *Textbook of Small Animal Surgery, 2nd Edition*, ed. D Slatter, pp. 325–340. W B Saunders, Philadelphia

Swaim SF and Henderson RA (1997) Wounds on limbs. In *Small Animal Wound Management, 2nd Edition*, ed. SF Swain and RA Henderson, pp. 311–318. Williams and Wilkins, Baltimore

CHAPTER TEN

Pedicled Muscle Flaps

Jonathan Chambers

INTRODUCTION

Local rotation of muscle is a powerful and versatile reconstructive tool for the veterinary surgeon and does not require special instrumentation or training. The most common indication for local transposition of muscle is to replace or augment tissues lost or severely damaged by trauma, surgical resection, radiation therapy or disease. The most important functions of the transposed muscle are:

- To restore a vascular covering for exposed ischaemic tissues
- To protect exposed tissues against infection and other environmental injury (e.g. desiccation, mechanical trauma).

Related benefits of the vascularized muscle are:

- Provision of substrates for wound healing (radiation injury)
- Bulk to fill dead space and restore cosmetic contours
- A vehicle for delivery of systemic antibiotics.

The transposed muscle provides an immediate vascularized surface to support transposed or grafted skin. Muscle flaps can also be used to patch defects in hollow organs.

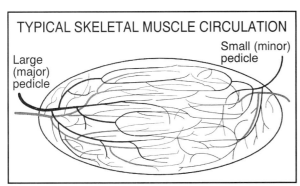

Figure 10.1: *Typical vascular supply to a skeletal muscle. Note that it is composed of a combination of large and small pedicles, and the pedicle systems often share small anastomotic channels at their borders.*

The ideal muscle for rotation is one that can be transposed to the injured area on a vascular pedicle that is constant in its location and has a reliable area of perfusion. But the muscle (or portion thereof) and its pedicle must also be distant enough from the injured area to ensure that neither is compromised by the disease process. The proposed muscle flap must be of appropriate dimensions for the task at hand. Excessive bulk can create mechanical and cosmetic problems, but atrophy secondary to denervation should be allowed for. The transposed muscle should be functionally expendable; rarely is this a dilemma because of the synergistic action of muscles.

RELATIONSHIPS OF PEDICLES AND PERFUSION

Most muscles are supplied by multiple vascular pedicles of varying size (Figures 10.1 and 10.2), but the transposed muscle must be sustained by a pedicle that has a consistent extramuscular location and distribution of its

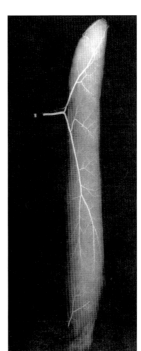

Figure 10.2: *Arteriogram of the cranial head of the sartorius muscle in the dog. Note that the muscle is supplied for the most part by a large pedicle from the superficial circumflex iliac artery and vein, but the proximal and distal ends are perfused by much smaller (minor) pedicles from the iliolumbar and descending genicular vessels, respectively.*

Reproduced from Chambers et al. (1990b) with permission.

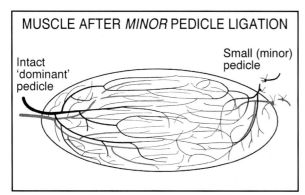

Figure 10.3: Perfusion of a muscle will be sustained throughout after ligation of minor pedicles because the remaining dominant pedicle is sufficiently large to maintain arterial and venous flow.

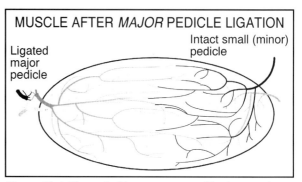

Figure 10.4: The probable consequence of basing muscle flap perfusion on a minor pedicle system. The volume of blood that can be forced through and returned via anastomotic channels is insufficient, and a large portion of muscle becomes severely ischaemic, if not necrotic.

intramuscular perfusion field. *Dominant* pedicles are those of sufficient size to perfuse the entire muscle flap predictably. Dominant pedicle systems have small intramuscular anastomoses with other *minor* pedicle systems serving the same muscle, and reverse flow through these 'choke' vessels will maintain perfusion throughout the entire muscle after the minor pedicles have been severed in preparation for transposition (Figure 10.3). Conversely, perfusion of entire muscle flaps through only minor pedicles *(distal flap)* is much less reliable (10.4). Some muscles, e.g. the semitendinosus, have co-dominant pedicles entering at both ends; thus, the entire muscle can be rotated in a wide arc proximally or distally, based on either of these pedicles.

Prospective flaps in dogs and cats have been proposed from anatomical studies, and perfusion studies have been done on a few. However, clinical trials involving numerous cases are lacking in veterinary surgery, and until such information is developed, caution is suggested against assumptions or extrapolations based solely on gross morphology.

GENERAL OPERATIVE TECHNIQUES

Several principles must be followed when transposing a pedicled muscle flap:

- The arc of rotation of a prospective muscle flap should be estimated based on an individual's standard landmarks to assure that the flap will reach the desired location; variations should be anticipated relative to extremes in body conformation. Optimal patient positioning should be planned for access to both donor and recipient sites
- It is wise to anticipate use of the entire muscle during exposure, dissection and mobilization. The muscle will contract as it, or its tendon, is sectioned, but it will relax back to at least the original length when its innervation is cut. Excessive length can be trimmed after transposition

- The dissection should start well away from the sustaining vascular pedicle, and gradually and meticulously approach it as the muscle becomes progressively more mobile
- Tendons of insertion and origin should be sectioned with impunity to relieve tension and increase the arc of rotation. Small branches of the sustaining artery to other muscles should also be ligated and sectioned to increase the length of the pedicle
- The safest method of routing the muscle flap to the recipient location is to create a liberal connecting incision. The pedicle and muscle must be observed closely during repositioning to guard against kinking, twisting or excessive tension. Gentle rotation or inversion of the flap will not usually create significant ischaemia. Intermuscular and subcutaneous tunnels can be created, but great care must be taken not to leave the muscle or pedicle constricted
- The flap and pedicle must be scrutinized during wound closure. The colour of the muscle is a relatively accurate measure of normal blood flow. Brisk haemorrhage from a cut edge or intraoperative monitoring with Doppler ultrasonography or oximetry are good measures of arterial perfusion but are poor indicators of the adequacy of venous drainage. It is especially important to realize this because technical errors may have a greater effect on the comparatively low pressure flow though the venous pedicle
- Tensionless closure of the skin over the transposed muscle is critical, and tension-relieving techniques, such as adjacent relaxing incisions, V–Y or Z plasties or axial pattern flaps, are used as necessary. If these procedures appear impractical or insufficient to alleviate pressure on the underlying muscle, the wound should be left open for immediate or delayed skin grafting. Well perfused muscle flaps serve as excellent beds for free split thickness skin grafts.

COMMON MUSCLE FLAPS

The pelvic limb

The superficial gluteal flap

Major pedicles: Caudal gluteal artery and vein proximally entering the deep face near the origin on the sacrum and sacrotuberous ligament.

Arc of rotation: Caudally to the anal sphincter.

Suggested indications for use: Dorsal augmentation of standard perineal hernia repair and perianal wounds.

Flap dissection: The tendon of insertion of the superficial gluteal muscle can be sectioned and rotated caudally with the muscle to augment the repair of perineal hernia. Sectioning of the originating tissues will increase the caudal mobilization but must be done with extreme care to avoid damaging the major pedicle(s).

The internal obturator flap

Major pedicle(s): Obturator branch of the medial circumflex femoral artery and vein, which enters the muscle after passing through the obturator foramen from ventral to dorsal at its cranial border.

Arc of rotation: Dorsomedially to the ipsilateral dorsal anal sphincter.

Suggested indications for use: Ventrolateral augmentation of standard perineal hernia repair.

Flap dissection: The internal obturator muscle is elevated subperiosteally from its origin on the caudal floor of the pelvis and the tendon of insertion may be cut to mobilize the flap. It is then everted medially and its borders sutured to surrounding tissues to repair perineal hernias (Figure 10.5). Care must be taken when elevating the cranial portion of the muscle and sectioning the tendon of insertion to avoid damage to the major vascular pedicle.

The cranial sartorius flap

Major pedicle: All of the muscle except the most proximal and distal tips is supplied by a pedicle of the superficial circumflex iliac artery and vein, which splits into proximally and distally directed branches before entering the caudal border of the muscle at the junction of the proximal and middle thirds (see Figure 10.1). The blood supply to the single sartorius muscle in the cat is similar to that to the cranial sartorius in the dog and can thus be used as a flap in the same fashion.

Arc of rotation: The distal end of the muscle can be rotated to the lateral thigh or hip, or the proximal end can be inverted on to the hip region. The distal tip of the muscle will reach the midline dorsally and the umbilicus cranially in most dogs.

Suggested indications for use:

- Pressure sores
- To fill dead space left by traumatic injuries or surgical resections in the regions of the greater trochanter and tuber ischium (Figure 10.6)
- Repair of caudal abdominal and femoral hernias
- Repair of rupture of the prepubic tendon.

Flap dissection: The caudal arc of rotation can be increased by dissecting the superficial circumflex pedicle towards the femoral artery and vein and dividing small branches to other muscles such as the caudal sartorius and tensor fasciae latae. Additional length can also be attained by passing the muscle beneath the tensor fasciae latae muscle; this will be required in most dogs to reach the tuber ischium.

The caudal sartorius flap

Pedicles: The caudal sartorius muscle is segmentally supplied by a series of relatively small pedicles distributed along its length, with intramuscular anastomoses between adjacent pedicle fields.

Flap development and use: Although there is little doubt that isolated segments of the muscle can be transposed locally, it has been suggested that the entire

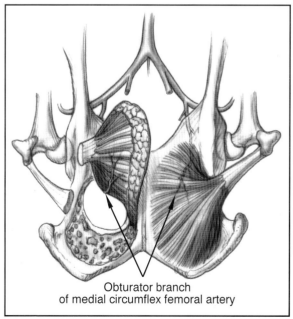

Obturator branch
of medial circumflex femoral artery

Figure 10.5: The internal obturator muscle flap, as elevated and inverted, based on the obturator branch of the medial circumflex femoral artery and vein to repair a perineal hernia.

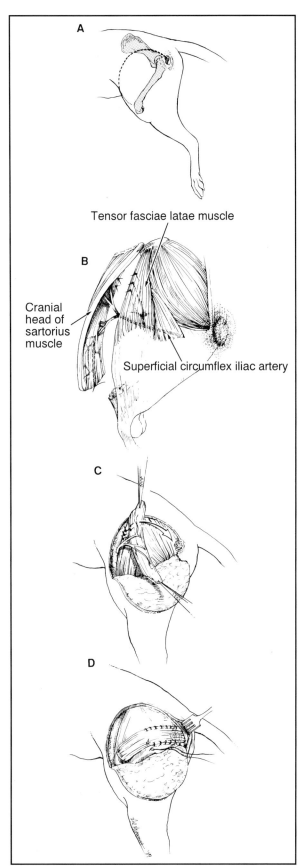

muscle can be transposed based on the more distal pedicle(s). This then requires that perfusing blood to the proximal portion of the muscle crosses one or more perfusion fields. Although this perfusion via minor pedicles is theoretically possible, caution is advised if robust perfusion to a recipient area is required.

The rectus femoris flap

Major pedicle: A single branch of the lateral circumflex femoral artery and vein, which enters the proximal end of the muscle on the caudal surface.

Arc of rotation: The distal end of the rectus femoris muscle can be rotated to the lateral thigh and hip regions.

Suggested indications for use:

- Pressure sores
- To fill dead space left by traumatic injuries or surgical resections in the adjacent regions of the thigh and greater trochanter

Flap alternatives: The rectus femoris flap is comparatively robust, and offers nothing over the cranial sartorius if it is available.

The semitendinosus flap

Major pedicles: Co-dominant pedicles of the caudal gluteal and distal caudal femoral vessels which enter the proximal and distal ends. respectively, along the cranial border (Figure 10.7); either pedicle system will perfuse to the entire muscle.

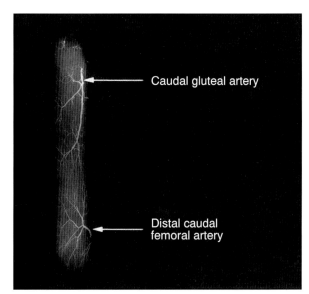

Figure 10.6: *Approach, elevation and eversion of the cranial sartorius muscle, based on the superficial circumflex iliac pedicle, to cover a pressure ulcer or repair a wound over the greater trochanter or tuber ischium.*

Reproduced from Chambers et al. (1990b) with permission.

Figure 10.7: *Blood supply to the semitendinosus muscle in the dog. Pedicles of approximately equal size enter at each end, and either will sustain flow for the entire length of muscle via the anastomotic network.*

Reproduced from Chambers and Rawlings (1991) with permission.

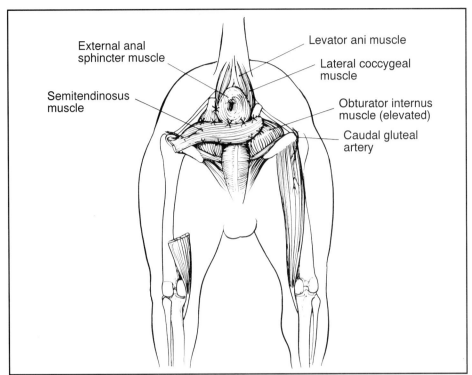

External anal
sphincter muscle

Semitendinosus
muscle

Levator ani muscle

Lateral coccygeal
muscle

Obturator internus
muscle (elevated)

Caudal gluteal
artery

Figure 10.8: Transposition of the semitendinosus muscle, based on the proximal caudal gluteal pedicle, to aid in the repair of complicated perineal hernia.

Reproduced from Chambers and Rawlings (1991) with permission.

Arc of rotation: Dorsally to just beyond the midline; cranially to the junction of the iliac body and wing; caudomedially to the contralateral tuber ischium; distally to the tarsus.

Suggested indications for use:

- The distal end can be rotated to surround the anus for repair of wounds or complicated perineal hernias (Figure 10.8). This flap is particularly useful for repair of perineal hernias with large ventral components, and those for which either the internal obturator or superficial gluteal flaps have failed
- Wounds over the crus can be repaired, and exposed tibia covered by a semitendinosus flap based on the distal pedicle.

Flap alternatives: The semitendinosus is a rather robust flap for transposition to the crus, and the cranial tibial or lateral gastrocnemius flaps should be considered as alternatives.

Cranial border of the lateral head of the gastrocnemius muscle

Major pedicle: A long pedicle of the popliteal vessels, which courses superficially from proximal to distal.

Arc of rotation: Adjacent areas of the proximal crus.

Suggested indications for use: Wounds adjacent to the stifle.

Cranial tibial flap

Pedicles: Segmental branches of the cranial tibial artery and vein.

Arc of rotation: Adjacent areas of the mid and distal crus.

Suggested indications for use: Avulsion wounds of the crus, especially open tibial fractures.

Flap dissection: The distal end of the cranial tibial muscle can be transposed locally on a short pedicle (Figure 10.9). Other isolated portions can presumably be transposed, based on their respective pedicles, but no clinical trials have been reported.

Muscles of the trunk, thoracic limb, head and neck

Rectus abdominus flap

Major pedicles: Co-dominant end pedicles from the cranial and caudal epigastric vessels, respectively.

Arc of rotation: Adjacent areas of the trunk.

Suggested indications for use: Reconstruction of wounds or replacement of resected portions of the body wall.

Flap alternatives: Cranial portion of the external abdominal oblique muscle, which is thinner and more pliable.

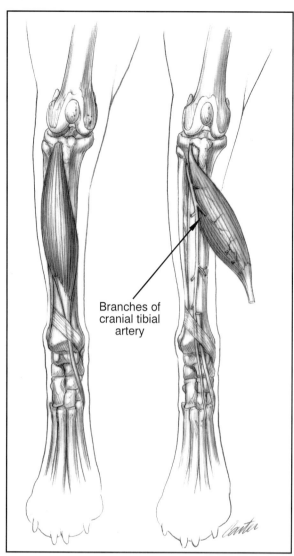

Figure 10.9: Transposition of the distal end of the cranial tibial muscle to cover adjacent wounds of the crus.

Cranial portion of external abdominal oblique muscle

Major pedicle: A pedicle of the cranial abdominal artery and vein.

Arc of rotation: Adjacent portions of the trunk wall; medial to the midline.

Suggested indications for use:

- Reconstruction of wounds
- Replacement of resected portions of the body wall
- Augmentation in repair of complex diaphragmatic hernias.

Flap alternatives – Rectus abdominus.

Latissimus dorsi flap

Major pedicle: A large branch of the thoracodorsal artery and vein, which enters the deep face near the junction of the cranial and middle thirds.

Arc of rotation: Adjacent areas of the thoracic wall; cranially to the lateral shoulder and brachial regions; distally to the proximal antebrachium; medially (intrathoracic) to the opposite chest wall.

Suggested indications for use:

- To cover defects left by tumour resection (Figure 10.10)
- Patching of intrathoracic leaks (lung, trachea, oesophagus)
- Augmentation of myocardial blood supply and function.

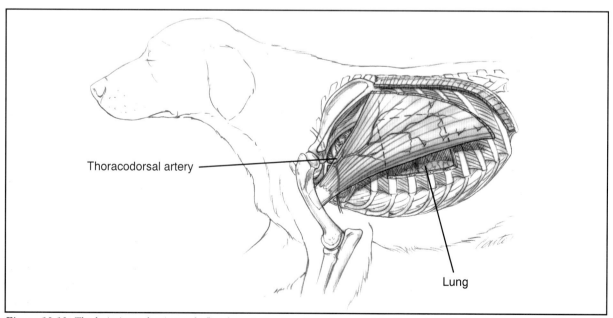

Figure 10.10: The latissimus dorsi muscle flap for rotation to adjacent areas of the thoracic wall, shoulder, or arm, or for intrathoracic transposition.

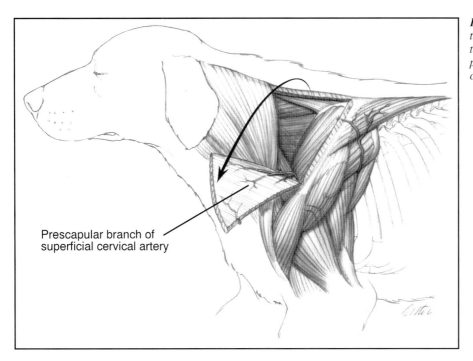

Figure 10.11: Transposition of the cervical portion of the trapezius muscle, based on pedicles from the superficial cervical artery and vein.

Prescapular branch of superficial cervical artery

Flap dissection: The latissimus dorsi muscle is released from its segmental attachments to the ribs.

Cervical portion of the trapezius muscle

Major pedicle: Branches of the prescapular division of the superficial cervical artery and vein, which enter the midcranial border close together (Figure 10.11).

Arc of rotation: The muscle can be rotated cranially on to the adjacent neck by inversion; distally on to the shoulder and brachium.

Suggested indications for use: Wounds about the neck, shoulder or arm.

Flap alternatives: Caudal portions of the sternocephalicus, sternothyroideus or sternohyoideus muscles.

Deep pectoral muscle (craniodorsal third)

Major pedicle: A pedicle of the lateral thoracic artery and vein, which enters cranially.

Arc of rotation: Adjacent areas of the trunk and neck.

Suggested indications for use: Wound reconstruction.

Deep pectoral muscle (caudoventral third)

Pedicles: A series of pedicles of the internal thoracic vessels, which enter along the sternal border.

Arc of rotation: Adjacent areas of the trunk; on to and across the ventral midline.

Suggested indications for use: Wound reconstruction, especially open injuries to the sternum.

Flap development: Distinct anastomoses between the internal thoracic and lateral thoracic pedicle systems have been identified, but it is unknown whether the entire deep pectoral muscle will survive on either pedicle system, as in man.

Humeral head of the flexor carpi ulnaris muscle

Major pedicles: A consistent pedicle of the caudal interosseous vessels, which enters on the deep face near the tendon of insertion on the accessory carpal bone (Figure 10.12). Intramuscular branches anastomose with branches of the ulnar and deep antebrachial vessels and mid muscle.

Arc of rotation: Adjacent areas of the distal antebrachium and carpus; distally to the metacarpal–phalangeal junction.

Suggested indications for use: Avulsion wounds, especially open fractures of the distal antebrachium, carpus and manus.

Flap dissection: The muscle can be rotated or inverted in either direction around the distal forearm or carpus to cover the more problematical surfaces.

Ulnaris lateralis flap

Pedicles: A *consistent* pedicle of the cranial interosseous artery and vein, which enters on the deep face proximally. An *inconsistent* pedicle of the caudal interosseous artery and vein, which enters the deep face near the musculotendinous junction.

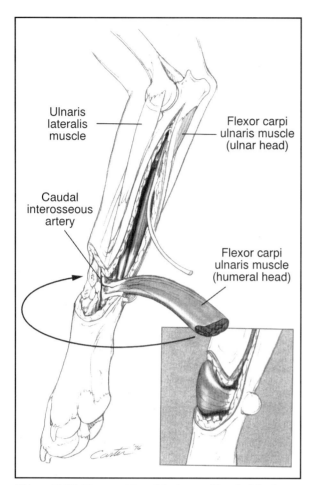

Figure 10.12: *Transposition of the humeral head of the flexor carpi ulnaris muscle, based on its distal interosseous pedicle.*

Reproduced from Chambers et al. (1998) with permission.

Arc of rotation: Adjacent areas of the antebrachium.

Suggested indication(s) for use: Wound reconstruction, especially coverage of severe open fractures of the proximal and mid antebrachium.

Flap development: The ulnaris lateralis is one of several antebrachial muscles that can be elevated on relatively short proximal pedicles and advanced to immediately adjacent areas. The ulnaris lateralis has been proposed for use distally in much the same way as the humeral head of the flexor carpi ulnaris, but caution is advised because the caudal interosseus pedicle is not identifiable in all specimens.

Flap alternative: Humeral head of the flexor carpi ulnaris muscle.

Caudal portions of the sternocephalicus, sternothyroideus, and sternohyoideus muscles

Major pedicle: Ascending branch of the superficial cervical artery and vein, which courses along and provides pedicles into the dorsal borders (Figure 10.13).

Arc of rotation: Adjacent areas of the caudal neck.

Suggested indication(s) for use:

- Repair wounds
- Patch and cover defects in viscera such as the oesophagus and trachea.

Flap dissection: These three muscles, especially the sternothyroideus and sternohyoideus, intimately share the ramifications of their caudal pedicles, and it may be easier and safer to transpose them as a unit.

Flap alternative: Cervical portion of the trapezius muscle.

Cranial portions of the sternocephalicus, sternothyroideus and sternohyoideus muscles

Major pedicle: The cranial thyroid artery and vein (see Figure 10.13).

Arc of rotation: Adjacent areas of the cranial neck and head.

Suggested indications for use: Patching and covering defects of the cranial oesophagus, trachea and larynx.

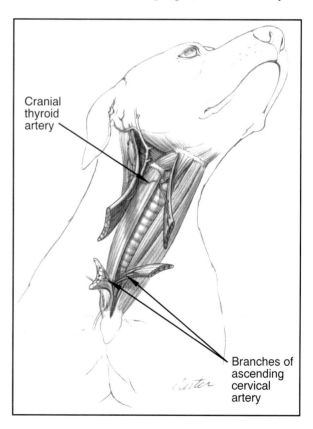

Figure 10.13: *Vascular supply to the sternocephalicus, sternothyroideus and sternohyoideus muscles. The cranial or caudal portions of these muscles can be transposed to adjacent areas, based on their respective pedicles.*

Flap dissection: Small intramuscular anastomotic branches have been identified at the mid portion of these muscles between the cranial thyroid and ascending cervical pedicle systems. If the perfusion across these 'choke' vessels is sufficient, then the entire length of these muscles could be transposed to reconstruct oral and nasal tissues, but this has yet to be investigated.

Temporalis flap

Major pedicles: Branches of the superficial and deep temporalis vessels with arborization parallel to the muscle fasciculi.

Arc of rotation: Immediately adjacent areas.

Suggested indications for use: Cosmetic and functional reconstruction of the orbit and paranasal sinuses.

Flap dissection: The overlying fascia is included in the flap to avoid damage to the superficial pedicles. Facial release and resection of orbital ligament and cranial zygoma facilitate cranial mobilization of the flap.

REFERENCES AND FURTHER READING

Alexander LG, Pavletic MM and Engler ST (1991) Abdominal wall reconstruction with a vascular external abdominal oblique myofascial flap. *Veterinary Surgery* **20**, 379-384

Basher AWP and Presnell KR (1987) Muscle transposition as an aid in covering traumatic tissue defects over the canine tibia. *Journal of the American Animal Hospital Association* **23**, 617-628

Chambers JN, Purinton PT, Allen SW and Moore JL (1990a) Identification and anatomical categorization of the vascular patterns to the pelvic limb muscles of dogs. *American Journal of Veterinary Research* **51**, 305-313.

Chambers JN, Purinton PT, Allen SW, Schneider TA and Smith JD (1998) A flexor carpi ulnaris (humeral head) muscle flap for reconstruction of distal forelimb injuries in dogs. *Veterinary Surgery* **27**, 342-347

Chambers JN, Purinton PT, Moore JL and Allen SW (1990b) Treatment of trochanteric ulcers with cranial sartorius and rectus femoris muscle flaps. *Veterinary Surgery* **19**, 424-428

Chambers JN and Rawlings CA (1991) Applications of a semitendinosus muscle flap in 2 dogs. *Journal of the American Veterinary Medical Association* **199**, 84-86

Gregory CR and Gourley IM (1991) Identification of muscle flaps in small animals. *Microsurgery* **12**, 136-139

Hardie EM, Kolata RJ, Earley TD, Rawlings CA and Gorgaz EJ (1983) Evaluation of internal obturator muscle transposition in treatment of perineal hernia in dogs. *Veterinary Surgery* **12**, 69-72

Pavletic MM (1990) Introduction to myocutaneous and muscle flaps. *Veterinary Clinics of North America: Small Animal Practice* **20**, 127-146

Pavletic MM (1993) Myocutaneous flaps and muscle flaps. In: *Atlas of Small Animal Reconstructive Surgery,* ed. MM Pavletic pp. 310-323. Lippincott, Philadelphia

Philibert D and Fowler JD (1996) Use of muscle flaps in reconstructive surgery. *Compendium of Continuing Education for the Practicing Veterinarian* **18**, 395-404

Philibert D, Fowler JD and Clapson JB (1991) The anatomical basis for a trapezius muscle flap in dogs. *Veterinary Surgery* **21**, 429-434

Purinton PT, Chambers JN and Moore JL (1992) Identification and categorization of the vascular patterns to muscles of the thoracic limb, thorax, and neck of dogs. *American Journal of Veterinary Research* **53**, 1435-1445

Sylvestre AM, Weinstein MJ, Popovitch CA and Brockman DJ (1997) The sartorius muscle flap in the cat: an anatomical study and two case reports. *Journal of the American Animal Hospital Association* **33**, 91-96

Tomlinson J and Presnell KR (1981) Use of the temporalis muscle flap in the dog. *Veterinary Surgery* **10**, 77-79

Weinstein MJ, Pavletic MM and Boudrieau RJ (1988) Caudal sartorius muscle flap in the dog. *Veterinary Surgery* **17**, 203-210

CHAPTER ELEVEN

Reconstructive Microsurgery

David Fowler

INTRODUCTION

The term microsurgery simply implies the use of magnification at some point during an operative procedure. The use of operating loupes and surgical microscopes has been commonplace in human neurosurgery, ophthalmic surgery and reconstructive surgery for decades.

Microvascular free tissue transfer refers to the dissection of an 'island' of tissue based on a feeding artery and vein, complete transection of the tissue from its donor site, transfer of the tissue to a recipient wound bed and revascularization of the tissue through microvascular anastomosis of the donor artery and vein to an appropriately sized recipient artery and vein. Tissues transferred in this manner are referred to as microvascular free tissue transfers, free flaps, microvascular free flaps or autogenous vascularized grafts.

Experience with microvascular free tissue transfer is limited in veterinary surgery. Fewer than one hundred procedures, using fewer than ten different flap designs, have been reported. Despite this fact, the utility of microvascular free tissue transfer for one-stage reconstruction of difficult problems has been established. Early reconstruction of traumatic tissue loss, using vascularized tissue, is feasible, as is functional and cosmetic reconstruction after ablative cancer surgery.

Any tissue, or combination of tissues, may be used in the development of a microvascular free flap, as long as it meets several criteria:

- The tissue must be nourished by a single source artery and drained by a single vein; generally the artery and vein parallel one another, although this is not an absolute requirement for a successful flap
- The source artery and vein must be of sufficient size to accommodate successful microvascular anastomosis; vessels less than 1 mm in diameter show progressively increased rates of thrombosis at the anastomosis
- The donor tissue must be dispensable. Reconstructive microsurgery has been referred to as 'the art of robbing Peter to pay Paul'; it is essential to ensure that 'Peter' will not miss the substance of which he is being robbed

- The tissue flap and its associated vessels should be relatively easy to identify and dissect.

Microvascular free flaps are identified according to the tissue type(s) included within the flap. Commonly used tissues include free cutaneous flaps, muscle flaps, omental flaps, bowel flaps and vascularized bone grafts. Combinations of tissues may also be incorporated into flap designs, resulting in the formation of myocutaneous flaps, myo-osseous flaps, osteomusculocutaneous flaps, etc. Free flaps are further identified according to the specific source of tissue. Examples include the trapezius muscle flap, the latissimus dorsi myocutaneous flap, the cranial abdominal myoperitoneal flap and the free vascularized ulnar bone graft.

The overall success rate reported for veterinary microvascular free tissue transfer is approximately 93%. This compares quite favourably with reported success rates in people. Training in microvascular technique is becoming relatively commonplace in veterinary surgical training programmes, and microvascular reconstructive procedures are being performed in several veterinary referral centres. Increasing levels of experience will undoubtedly result in the use of microvascular tissue transfer as the reconstructive technique of first choice for complex and difficult reconstructive problems.

MICROVASCULAR TECHNIQUE

Instrumentation
Equipment required for microvascular free tissue transfer is not extensive, but is relatively expensive. The following are basic requirements.

Operating microscope
An operating microscope (Figure 11.1) is essential for successful repair of the small vessels generally used in microvascular reconstruction (1-2 mm diameter). The microscope should have a foot control for adjustment of coarse focus, fine focus and magnification, leaving the surgeon's hands free for surgical manipulations. The range of magnification used varies from approximately 5X to 30X. It is also beneficial to have a foot-controlled 'X-Y axis' on the microscope. This

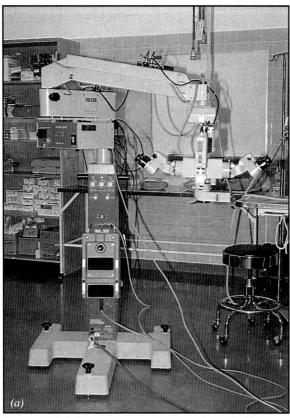

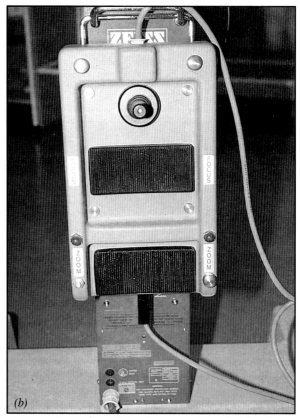

Figure 11.1: (a) An operating microscope is needed for successful microvascular surgery. This microscope is fitted with a 'beam splitter', allowing two surgeons to view the same surgical field with stereoscopic vision. (b) A foot pedal control facilitates adjustment of the microscope, leaving the surgeon's hands free. This foot pedal has adjustments for zoom, focus, and an 'X–Y' axis that allows repositioning of the field of vision.

allows the surgeon to move the head of the operating microscope in two planes and is useful when dissecting along the length of a vessel or shifting between vessels. Ideally, the operating microscope has a beam-splitter that provides an identical stereoscopic visual field to two surgeons. Although microvascular anastomosis may be accomplished by one surgeon, it is greatly facilitated by a second.

Surgical instruments
The following instruments are used (Figure 11.2):

- Jeweller's forceps are required for manipulation of small vessels. Number 3 and number 5 jeweller's forceps are generally of greatest use. Number 3 forceps are used for handling of the vessel during initial dissection. Number 5 forceps are used for final dissection, during anastomosis, or for handling very small vessels. Curved or angled jeweller's forceps are useful for grasping the 'back-side' of the vessel wall during vascular dissection
- Vessel dilators are similar to jeweller's forceps, but have a blunted tip to help prevent intimal injury. Vessel dilators are inserted into the vessel lumen prior to anastomosis and are used to dilate the end of the vessel gently, thereby facilitating handling and suturing of the vessel end

- Very fine microsurgical scissors are required for adventitial dissection and vessel transection. It is beneficial to have both straight and curved scissors to facilitate vascular dissection in all planes
- Both straight and curved microsurgical needle drivers are available, with varying tip dimensions.

Very small suture material and needles are also recommended for microvascular anastomosis (Figure 11.2).

Microvascular approximating clamps
Microvascular approximating clamps (Figure 11.3) may have several different features, depending upon the specific use and the preference of the surgeon. Approximating clamps are used to stabilize vessel ends in approximation, and to block blood flow in the vessel and haemorrhage at the site during anastomosis:

- Double clamps consist of two clamps (one for each vessel end) connected on a sliding bar. After placing the donor and recipient vessel ends into opposing clamps, the clamps are adjusted on the sliding bar to bring the vessels into approximation

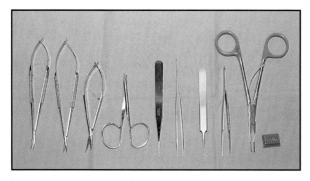

Vessel diameter	Suture size	Needle size
< 1 mm	11-0	50 µm
1-2 mm	10-0	70 or 100 µm
> 2 mm	9-0 or 10-0	100 µm

Figure 11.2: Fine microsurgical instruments are required for atraumatic handling and dissection of small vessels. An assortment of fine adventitial scissors, vessel dilators, jeweller's forceps and vascular clips is shown. Fine suture materials and needles are also required: the recommended sizes are shown in the table.

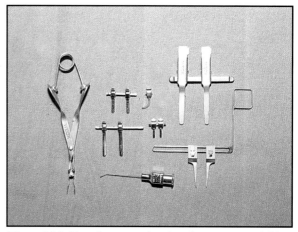

Figure 11.3: Vascular approximating clamps are available in various sizes and as single or double clamps. It is important that clamp size is matched to vessel size to ensure security of the vessel during anastomosis, but to avoid vessel injury from excessive clamp pressure.

- Double clamps can be provided with a wire frame. Long suture ends from previously placed sutures may be affixed to the wire frame to gain additional stability and to provide specific positioning of the vessel in preparation for the next suture. These are generally reserved for situations where an assistant surgeon is not available
- Single clamps are used to control haemorrhage temporarily after vessel transection, but prior to anastomosis
- Microvascular clamps are available in varying sizes. Each size will accommodate a specific range of vessel diameters. It is important that an appropriately sized clamp is used. Too large a clamp will produce a crush injury, while too small a clamp will allow the vessel end to slip.

Flap dissection

It is advantageous, although not absolutely necessary, to have two surgical teams during microvascular free tissue transfer. One surgical team harvests the flap (Figure 11.4) while the second surgical team exposes recipient vessels and prepares the wound bed for transfer. The use of two surgical teams will significantly reduce operating time. When only one experienced team is available, the flap is dissected first, leaving the vascular pedicle intact. Following preparation of the recipient site, the vascular pedicle of the flap is transected and transferred.

It is imperative that the surgeon understands the vascular anatomy of the flap to be dissected. Many flaps have been identified and described in the veterinary literature, and descriptions of new flaps will undoubtedly follow. It must be remembered that microvascular free flaps are totally dependent upon a single vascular source for survival after transfer, and that inadvertent damage to the vascular supply during flap dissection can have disastrous consequences.

Flap dissection is begun distant to the vascular pedicle. The tissues should be handled gently. When multiple tissue planes are present, such as in a myocutaneous flap, sutures are placed, as needed, to prevent shearing of tissue planes during dissection. Vascular branches that are isolated distant to the vascular pedicle may be controlled by traditional ligature or cautery techniques. As dissection approaches the vascular pedicle, great care must be taken to ensure a non-traumatic dissection of the vessels. Small vascular branches arising from the vascular pedicle may be carefully ligated using 9-0 or 10-0 suture material. Small vascular haemostatic clips may be used on larger vascular branches. Bipolar cautery may be used cautiously to coagulate vascular branches, but cautery must be performed sufficiently distant to the parent artery that endothelial thermal injury is avoided.

The vascular pedicle is 'skeletonized' after its identification, by dissecting along the vessels' adventitial surfaces. The full thickness of the vessel wall must not be grasped during manipulation since this will result in injury to the intimal surface. Instead, jeweller's forceps are used to grasp only the adventitial surface and gently elevate the vessel to allow dissection. The artery and vein are dissected to a length beyond that estimated to be required to ensure excess length of the vascular pedicle after transfer to the recipient site. The vessels are then trimmed to an appropriate length at the time of anastomosis. Once vascular dissection is complete, the flap is wrapped in moist sponges. The vascular pedicle should not be transected until the recipient site is prepared in order to minimize flap ischaemic time.

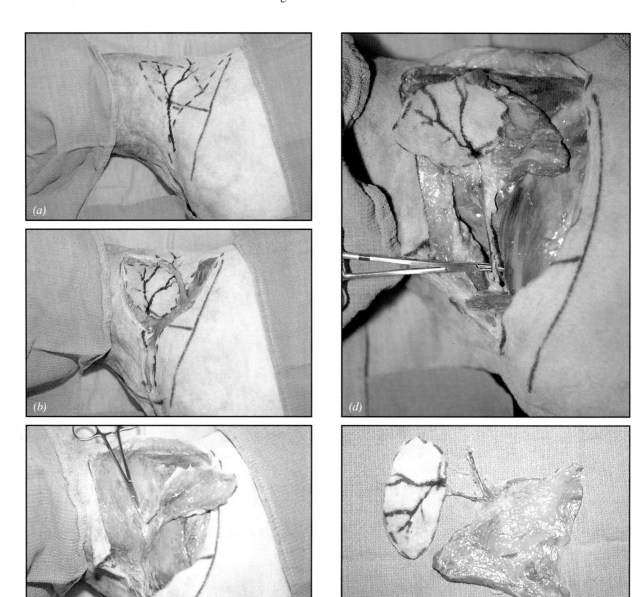

Figure 11.4: *The surgical approach to flap harvest. (a) All pertinent anatomical landmarks are identified prior to incision. Landmarks and proposed incision for harvest of the trapezius myocutaneous flap are indicated. (b) Skin incision is made and small bleeding vessels are carefully controlled using electrocautery. Dissection is begun distant from and continued towards major vascular pedicles. (c) Vascular pedicles must be identified and preserved during flap dissection. (d) The vascular pedicle is skeletonized after its identification. As much length of the vascular pedicle as possible should be harvested. (e) Final appearance of the dissected myocutaneous flap, showing the vascular pedicle and its associated muscle and skin territories.*

Recipient site preparation

Preparation of the recipient wound bed is extremely important. Free flaps are not a solution to suboptimal wound management. Wound beds must be free of ongoing tissue necrosis and active infection. Infected wounds, especially those with osteomyelitis, may be managed with microvascular free flaps as part of a one-stage operation, but thorough debridement of all infected tissue remains a necessity (Figure 11.5).

Consideration must be given to selecting an appropriate recipient artery and vein to be used in revascularizing the free flap. This requires a thorough knowledge of regional vascular anatomy. In cases of severe and extensive trauma, preoperative angiography is indicated to document the integrity and location of regional vessels. There are several criteria that must be considered when selecting an appropriate recipient artery and vein:

- Recipient vessels should be dissected outside the margins of the 'zone of trauma' to ensure the use of vessels without pre-existing intimal injury
- Recipient vessels must approximate the diameter of flap vessels when performing end-to-end anastomosis
- A size discrepancy of approximately 1.5:1 may be accommodated fairly easily when performing end-to-end anastomosis, but a greater size discrepancy leads to an increasing incidence of thrombosis

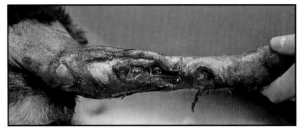 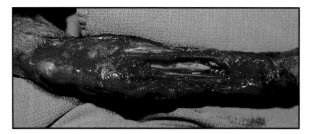

Figure 11.5: Necrotic and heavily contaminated tissue must be excised prior to wound reconstruction. Aggressive debridement and open wound management has converted this heavily contaminated forelimb injury to a clean contaminated state over a 3-day period.

- Recipient vessels should be larger than donor vessels when performing end-to-side anastomosis
- Incisions used to access recipient vessels are planned such that suture lines will not directly overlie the vascular pedicles. Curved incisions, resulting in the formation of a skin flap over the recipient vessels, are generally indicated
- It is important to consider flap location and the position of vascular pedicles prior to starting dissection of recipient vessels. Anticipation of the exact location where anastomosis will be performed will limit the amount of recipient vessel dissection that needs to be performed.

End-to-end anastomosis 'steals' the vascular supply of the recipient artery from its terminal destination and diverts that blood supply into the microvascular free flap. This is an important consideration in situations involving compromised vascularity to structures distal to the reconstruction. In these instances, end-to-side anastomosis should be performed in order to ensure vascular integrity of distal structures (Figure 11.6).

End-to-end anastomosis
This technique is illustrated in Figure 11.7.

1. The donor and recipient vessels are placed into approximation, using a double microvascular approximating clamp, and the lengths of the dissected vessels are checked to ensure that they are not twisted or kinked. Excessive tension and vessel redundancy must be avoided. If vessels are too long, the vessels are transected at an appropriate length. Inadequate vessel length presents a more difficult problem. In this instance, the intervening space must be bridged using a vein graft
2. Once the vessel ends have been trimmed and placed into the approximating clamp, the clamps are adjusted along the slide bar such that the vessels are not quite in contact with one another. This allows for easy identification of the vessel lumen during suture placement, but prevents undue tension on the sutures while tying. Contrast background material is placed beneath the vessels to facilitate handling and visual identification

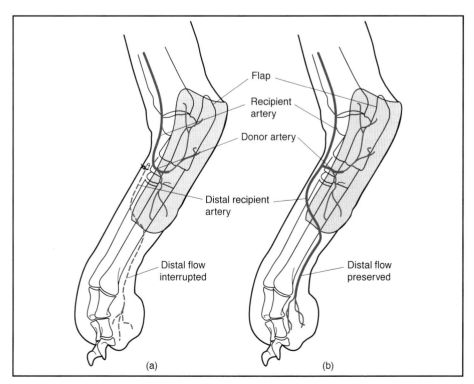

Figure 11.6: (a) End-to-end arterial anastomosis results in diversion of arterial flow away from distal structures normally nourished by the recipient artery. (b) End-to-side arterial anastomosis allows revascularization of the transferred tissue while maintaining distal arterial flow.

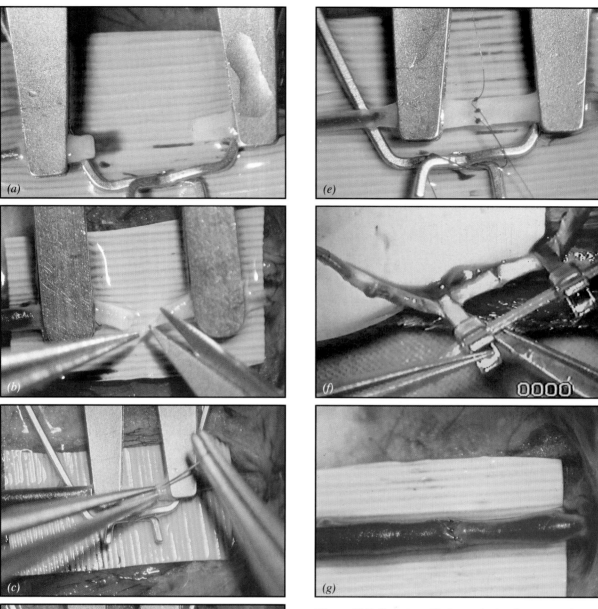

Figure 11.7: *Steps in achieving end-to-end anastomosis.*
(a) The recipient and donor vessel ends are placed into an
approximating clamp. Vessel ends are flushed with
heparinized saline solution (10 IU/ml) and the clamp is
adjusted to bring the vessel ends into approximation.
(b) Loose adventitial tissue is excised from the vessel ends.
(c) and (d) Simple interrupted sutures are placed at the 10
and 2 o'clock positions. Forceps are used to apply back
pressure during suture placement. The full thickness of the
vessel wall should never be grasped with forceps. (e) The
'front wall' of the anastomosis is completed. (f) The 'back
wall' is brought into view by inverting the approximating
clamp. (g) Closure is completed and the approximating
clamp is removed.

3. Adventitial tissue is extremely thrombogenic and must be dissected from the vessel ends to avoid its incorporation into the anastomosis. This is most easily accomplished by grasping the loose adventitial tissue with jeweller's forceps and placing traction on the vessel. The adventitial tissue is pulled beyond the level of the vessel end in a 'shirt-sleeve' fashion. The vessel end is easily identfed through the translucent adventitia, and the excess adventitia is amputated at the level of the vessel end. The adventitia is then allowed to retract back onto the vessel, leaving the terminal few millimetres of the vessel free of adventitia

4. After adventitial dissection, vessels are flushed with a heparin:saline solution, prepared at a concentration of 10 IU heparin per 1 ml saline, to remove debris and blood elements
5. The size of needle and suture material used is critical (see Figure 11.2b)
6. Several suturing techniques have been described for end-to-end anastomosis, but the 'front wall' technique is most commonly employed:
   - The vessel lumen is divided into thirds. With the 12 o'clock position defined as the centremost position of the superior vessel wall, simple interrupted sutures are placed at the 10 and 2 o'clock positions
   - Jeweller's forceps are used to place counter-pressure gently against the vessel wall during needle placement. The full thickness of the vessel wall should not be grasped since this will cause intimal injury at the anastomosis
   - A third simple interrupted suture is placed at the 12 o'clock position
   - Further sutures are placed as needed to complete apposition of the 'front wall'

- The microvascular approximating clamp is then turned over such that the previous 'back wall' is brought into the superior position. Previously placed sutures are inspected to ensure proper placement
- A simple interrupted suture is placed at the central point of the remaining defect, and the anastomosis is completed by placing additional simple interrupted sutures.

End-to-side anastomosis
This technique is illustrated in Figure 11.8.

1. End-to-side anastomosis is performed when dealing with a marked size discrepancy, the recipient vessel being larger than the donor vessel. Adventitial tissue is dissected from the donor vessel as described for end-to-end anastomosis and a single microvascular clamp is placed, if needed, across the donor vessel to facilitate handling and prevent passive efflux of blood from the vessel during anastomosis

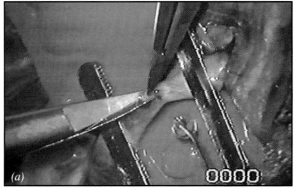
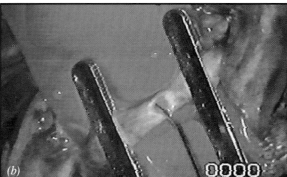
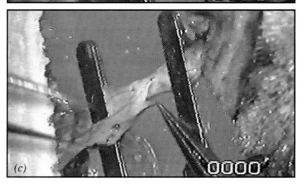
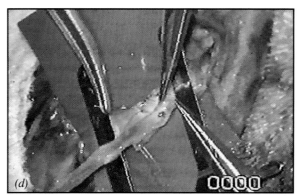
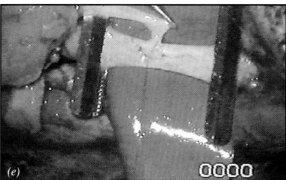

Figure 11.8: End-to-side anastomosis. (a) The recipient vessel is secured in a double approximating clamp. Adventitial tissue is dissected and an opening approximating the size of the donor vessel is made. (b) Blood is flushed from the recipient vessel using heparinized saline solution. (c) Simple interrupted sutures are placed at the 6 and 12 o'clock positions. (d) Retraction of the donor vessel in one direction facilitates closure of one side of the anastomosis. (e) Retraction in the opposite direction allows completion of the anastomosis.

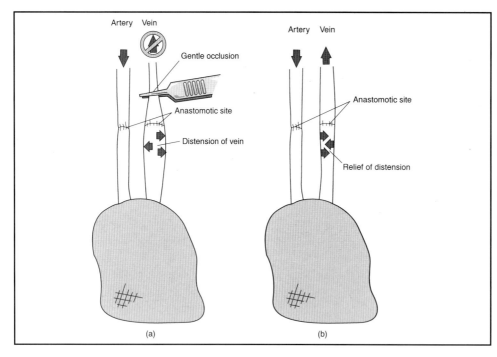

Figure 11.9: *The venous occlusion test is a safe and reliable method to assess patency of both the arterial and the venous anastomoses. (a) Gentle occlusion of the recipient vein 'downstream' from the anastomosis results in distension of the vein 'upstream'. Rapid distension reveals a patent arterial anastomosis. (b) Rapid relief of venous distension following release of the vein is compatible with a patent venous anastomosis.*

2. The recipient vessel wall is dissected free of adventitial covering for a length of several millimetres at the proposed site of anastomosis. A double microvascular approximating clamp is placed on to the recipient vessel, such that one clamp is situated proximal and one distal to the site of anastomosis

3. An opening must be made into the recipient vessel to accommodate the donor vessel. The size and precision of this opening is critical to the success of the anastomosis:
   - The vessel wall is grasped using jeweller's forceps and a full-thickness cut is made into the vessel at an angle of approximately 45 degrees using fine dissection scissors
   - The depth of the cut should be sufficient to result in an opening of approximately 50% of the size of that required
   - A matching cut is then made from the opposing side, and is planned such that the terminal ends of each cut meet precisely
   - The resulting opening will assume a round to oval configuration due to tensile forces from the vessel wall.

4. Heparinized saline solution is used to lavage blood elements and debris gently from the donor and recipient vessels

5. The donor vessel is brought into approximation with the recipient vessel and simple interrupted sutures are placed at the 3 o'clock and 9 o'clock positions

6. A third suture is placed at the 12 o'clock position and interposing sutures are used to complete the anastomosis along one side of the vessel. Retraction of the donor vessel by the assistant facilitates suture placement

7. Finally, a suture is placed at the 6 o'clock position, and the anastomosis is completed.

Assessing patency

The order of vascular repair, artery first or vein first, is largely a matter of personal preference. Flow should not be re-established through either anastomosis until both are completed. At that time, the venous anastomosis should be released, followed by the arterial anastomosis. The order of clamp release is donor vein, recipient vein, donor artery and, finally, recipient artery.

Thrombosis at the anastomotic site, resulting from faulty technique, is usually apparent within 15 minutes of re-establishing blood flow. Blood flow should be confirmed a few minutes after clamp release, and again at 15 minutes after clamp release. Several methods have been described for this purpose. Simple visual inspection of the vessel is not a reliable indicator of blood flow since longitudinal pulsation may be seen in a thrombosed artery.

One of the simplest reliable tests for vascular patency is the venous occlusion test (Figure 11.9):

- The vein is visualized under magnification
- Jeweller's forceps are used to occlude the recipient vein gently, immediately 'downstream' from the anastomosis
- Progressive venous distension 'upstream' from the occlusion indicates a patent arterial anastomosis
- Once venous engorgement is seen (this requires only a few seconds) the jeweller's forceps are released. Immediate relief of venous distension indicates a patent venous anastomosis.

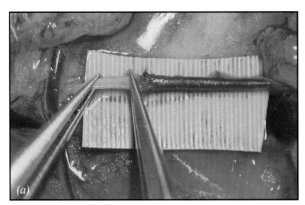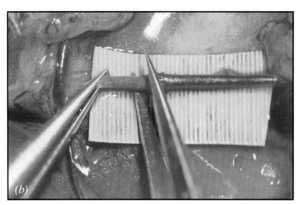

Figure 11.10: *The empty and refill test can be used to test both arterial and venous patency. (a) The vessel is grasped gently using two jeweller's forceps 'downstream' from the anastomosis. Blood is 'milked' from a vessel segment. (b) Release of the 'upstream' forceps should result in rapid refill of the emptied segment.*

A second commonly used patency test is the 'empty and refill' test (Figure 11.10), using two jeweller's forceps:

- The vessel is occluded with one pair of jeweller's forceps immediately 'downstream' from the anastomosis
- A second pair of jeweller's forceps is used to 'milk' blood gently from the vessel lumen, and subsequently occlude the vessel 1–2 cm further 'downstream'
- The 'upstream' forceps are released and the vessel is observed. Rapid refill of the emptied segment is indicative of a patent anastomosis.

Postoperative care

Astute postoperative care and monitoring are essential. Flaps are reliant upon the integrity of a single artery and vein for vascular flow. Restrictive bandages must be avoided and patient positioning must be planned to avoid compression of the vascular pedicle. The patient's hydration is maintained by provision of intravenous balanced electrolyte solutions or colloids. Flaps are kept warm by application of circulating warm water blankets, heat lamps, or loosely applied bandages.

Bandages are applied loosely to protect the flap from trauma or self-mutilation. A window is cut through the bandage to allow frequent visual inspection. Cutaneous flaps should maintain a pink appearance. Blanching of the flap is a possible indication of arterial insufficiency, while congestion and purplish discolouration is consistent with venous insufficiency. Brisk flow of bright red blood following pin-prick with a 20–22 gauge needle indicates adequate perfusion. Sluggish flow of dark blood is consistent with poor perfusion or arterial insufficiency. Transcutaneous doppler flow transducers may be used to verify flow through a superficially located arterial pedicle.

Early detection of failing flaps often leads to successful salvage. Re-exploration of the vascular pedicle is indicated at the first suggestion of poor perfusion. Corrective action depends on the specific cause of failure, but may necessitate repeat anastomosis, re-

location of vascular pedicles, or additional vascular dissection. Medicinal leeches may be used for the management of venous insufficiency in the presence of adequate arterial inflow.

Antithrombotic and anticoagulant drugs are not routinely recommended. Patency rates in excess of 95% are expected, given proper planning and meticulous technique. Antithrombotic agents are not a substitute for accurate surgical technique. In animals at risk of development of thrombosis, low-dose aspirin or systemic heparin therapy may be beneficial.

SPECIFIC FLAPS IN THE DOG AND CAT

Cutaneous flaps

Cutaneous angiosomes ('territories' of tissue that are supplied by a single source artery and vein) have been described thoroughly in the dog and cat and this information has been used for the development of large axial pattern skin flaps (see Chapter 8). These flaps may also be used for free microvascular transfer, assuming adequate size of the vascular pedicle for successful anastomosis. Vessel diameters for most described cutaneous flaps in dogs of average size approach 1–2 mm. The superficial cervical (omocervical) axial pattern flap, the caudal superficial epigastric axial pattern flap, and the saphenous fasciocutaneous conduit flap have been used clinically for microvascular transfer.

Detailed anatomical descriptions of flap dissection are given in Chapter 8. Two points are worth emphasizing here:

- The microvascular supply to axial pattern flaps, in areas where superficial cutaneous musculature exists, courses deep to this muscular layer. Dissection must, therefore, be performed deep to the superficial cutaneous musculature. For example, the cutaneous trunci muscle must be included with the dissection of the thoracodorsal cutaneous flap

- During flap dissection, there is a tendency for tensile or shearing forces to cause a separation between tissue layers. Placement of occasional simple interrupted sutures between cutaneous musculature, subcutaneous tissue and dermis helps to stabilize these tissues and prevent trauma to the microvasculature.

Footpad flaps

Footpads are specialized cutaneous/subcutaneous structures designed for resistance to weight-bearing stresses. Injury to large portions of the footpads inevitably results in compromised function. Reconstruction of such defects requires the use of 'like' tissue to replace lost tissue:

- The fifth digital footpad has been described as a microvascular free flap based on the deep plantar metatarsal artery IV and the superficial metatarsal vein IV
- The digital footpad and associated soft tissues are harvested following excision of the phalanges through a dorsal incision (Figure 11.11)
- Sensory re-innervation may be provided by repair of the deep plantar metatarsal nerve IV to an appropriate sensory nerve at the recipient site. However, the necessity of sensory re-innervation of transferred footpads has not been established.

The accessory carpal footpad has also been used as a microvascular free tissue transfer based on the caudal interosseous artery and the cephalic (Figure 11.12):

- A sensory branch of the ulnar nerve parallels the arterial pedicle through the carpal canal, and may be used for sensory re-innervation
- The carpal footpad is not situated in a weight-bearing position, but it shares the physical characteristics of a weight-bearing footpad. Loss of the carpal footpad is of no functional consequence.

Both the digital footpad and carpal footpad flaps are of limited size relative to most weight-bearing defects requiring reconstruction. Careful positioning of footpad tissue is required at the recipient site, to ensure fixation in a central weight-bearing position. Excessive shear forces and partial incisional dehiscence of the flap margins inevitably occur if the footpad becomes displaced (Figure 11.13). In the author's experience, several minor revisional procedures for flap repositioning are commonly required. Over time, the transferred footpads hypertrophy, thereby adopting a more functional weight-bearing role at the recipient site.

Muscle flaps

Muscle is probably the most useful of any single tissue used for wound reconstruction. It facilitates revascularization of ischaemic wound beds, delivers nutrients to the wound and decreases the incidence of significant wound complications, such as infection and delayed healing. Muscle flaps are generally quite easily dissected due to their enveloping fascial layers. Vascular pedicles are easily identified and protected. Most

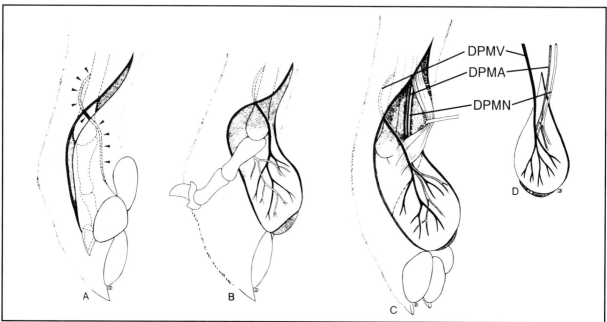

Figure 11.11: Harvest of the fifth digital footpad flap. (A) The incision is initiated laterally over the fifth metatarsal bone and curves distally to end on the dorsal aspect of the coronary band. (B) The phalangeal bones are dissected extraperiosteally. Care is necessary to avoid damage to neurovascular structures in the surrounding soft tissues. (C) The vascular pedicle, consisting of the superficial dorsal metatarsal vein (SDMV), the deep plantar metatarsal artery (DPMA) and deep plantar metatarsal nerve (DPMN), is identified. The broken line indicates the level of skin incision through the interdigital skin to complete flap formation. (D) Appearance of the dissected flap, as viewed from the deep surface.

(Reproduced with permission from Basher et al., 1990.)

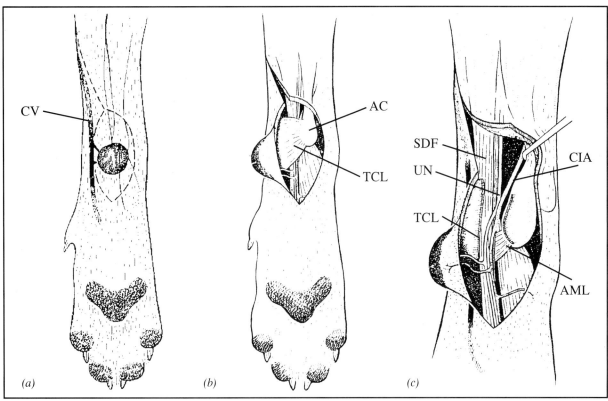

(a) *(b)* *(c)*

Figure 11.12: *Anatomical landmarks for dissection of the carpal footpad flap. (a) Circumferential skin incision around the footpad is extended proximally, parallel to the cephalic vein (CV). (b) Deep subcutaneous dissection is initiated from the lateral aspect until the small arterial branch to the footpad is identified. The accessory carpal bone (AC) and the transverse carpal ligament (TCL) are shown. (c) After dissection through the carpal canal, the caudal interosseous artery (CIA) and a superficial branch of the ulnar nerve (UN) are identified as they course between the transverse carpal ligament and the accessory metacarpeum ligament (AML). The pedicle closely parallels the tendon of the superficial digital flexor muscle (SDF). Venous drainage is provided by the cephalic vein.*

(Reproduced with permission from Moens and Fowler, 1997.)

muscles may be harvested with little resulting donor site morbidity. In nearly all instances, synergistic muscle groups adapt to the loss of a single muscle with little functional consequence. When muscle alone is used for reconstruction of wounds, overlying cutaneous resurfacing is accomplished by immediate placement of a full thickness skin graft on to the transferred muscle. The success of such grafts is consistently excellent.

The vascular supply to muscles may be divided into one of five basic types, based on the number and size of vascular pedicles nourishing the muscle. This classification system, and the specific vascular anatomy of commonly used muscles, is described in Chapter 10. Muscles with a type I, type II, or type V vascular pattern are preferred for microvascular transfer since their survival is expected, based entirely upon revascularization of only the dominant vascular pedicle. The trapezius muscle flap and the latissimus dorsi muscle flap are most commonly used for microvascular transfer.

Trapezius muscle flap

The cervical portion of the trapezius muscle has a type II vascular pattern, with the prescapular branch of the superficial cervical artery forming the dominant vascu-

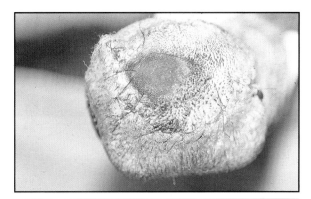

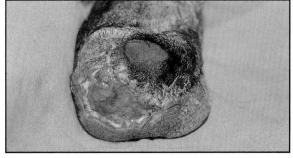

Figure 11.13: *Shear stresses acting upon weight-bearing incisions frequently result in partial dehiscence and flap migration. Minor revisional procedures are often required after footpad transfer.*

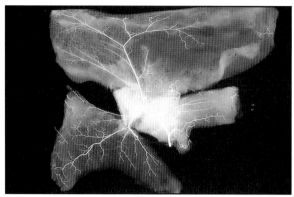

Figure 11.14: *Radiograph of the vascular territory of the prescapular branch of the superficial cervical artery. The vascular pedicle is in the centre. The trapezius muscle is shown in the lower left, a segment of the omotransversarius muscle in the centre, and the cutaneous territory in the upper portion.*

lar pedicle (Figure 11.14). Survival of the entire cervical portion of the trapezius muscle has been documented consistently based on this dominant pedicle:

1. Dissection of the trapezius muscle flap is performed through a curvilinear incision beginning approximately 2 cm cranial to the point of the shoulder, extending dorsally parallel to the scapular spine and curving cranially below the dorsal midline (Figure 11.15)

2. A flap of skin, subcutaneous tissue and superficial cutaneous musculature is elevated from the underlying trapezius muscle
3. The direct cutaneous branch of the superficial cervical artery (the vascular pedicle of the superficial cervical axial pattern skin flap) is identified and ligated as it exits the septum formed by the trapezius, the omotransversarius and the cleidocervicalis muscles
4. The cervical portion of the trapezius muscle is incised from its attachment to the scapular spine. Dorsal fascial attachments are incised and bleeding vessels are cauterized or ligated as required.
5. The muscle is gently elevated and several vascular branches extending to deep musculature are identified, ligated and transected. At this point the superficial cervical vascular system is readily visualized. In some dogs, the vessels adopt a course immediately beneath the body of the trapezius muscle; in others, the vessels parallel the cranial border of the trapezius muscle. Dissection in the latter group must be performed cautiously to preserve the integrity of the vascular pedicle
6. Dissection is continued towards the vascular pedicle, incising between the trapezius and cleidocervicalis muscles. One or two small vascular branches to the omotransversarius

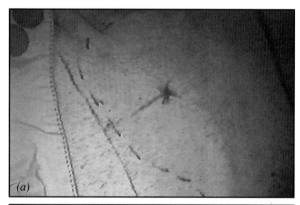

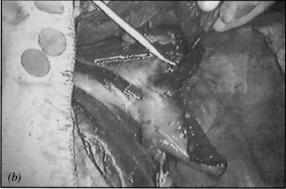

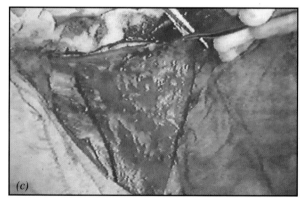

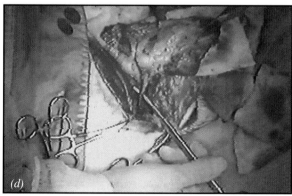

Figure 11.15: *Dissection of the trapezius muscle flap (see also Figure 11.4). (a) Anatomical landmarks identified include the scapular spine. The position of the direct cutaneous artery is marked with an X. The dashed line indicates the proposed incision. The dog's head is towards the upper right of the photograph. (b) Elevation of the trapezius muscle is begun along its scapular and dorsal fascial attachments. Vascular branches emanating from the parent pedicle are identified on the deep surface of the muscle. Several branches extending into the deep cervical musculature are ligated and divided. (c) After identification of the vascular pedicle, cranial and ventral dissection of the trapezius muscle is completed. (d) The vascular pedicle is skeletonized but not transected. Perfusion is maintained with the flap protected in moist sponges until the recipient site is prepared.*

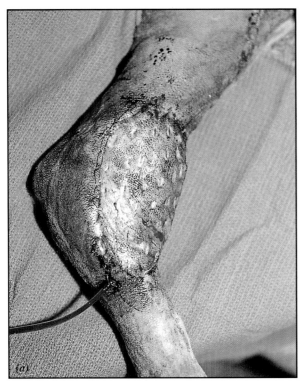 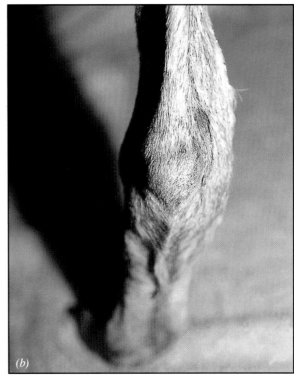

Figure 11.16: *Transferred muscle rapidly undergoes neurogenic atrophy. (a) Bulky appearance of a trapezius muscle transfer with overlying skin graft immediately after transfer. (b) Appearance of the same flap, in profile, 6 weeks after transfer.*

muscle are identified, ligated and transected, completing elevation of the trapezius muscle

7. The artery and vein are then skeletonized for a length of at least 2–3 cm. The prescapular lymph node is intimately associated with the vascular pedicle and may be incorporated in the dissection, or cautiously dissected free of the vascular pedicle. Inclusion of the lymph node in the dissection will result in a bulky vascular pedicle and may cause difficulty in closing incisions overlying the vascular pedicle at the recipient site.

The trapezius muscle is broad and flat and, therefore, lends itself well to the cosmetic reconstruction of many wounds. The bulk of the flap also rapidly diminishes due to denervation atrophy (Figure 11.16). Vascular density of muscle flaps has been shown to be maintained despite progressive muscle atrophy.

Significant donor site morbidity includes immediate postoperative pain and the development of seromas. Narcotic analgesics are generally required for 24–48 hours, followed by the administration of NSAIDs for 3–5 days. Seroma formation occurs to variable extents in all trapezius flap donor sites. Prophylactic drainage, using either a closed suction or passive system, should be provided.

Latissimus dorsi muscle flap

The latissimus dorsi muscle is a large, relatively flat muscle. It is used commonly for the reconstruction of large soft tissue deficits in people, and has been used to a limited extent in dogs and cats. It has a type V

vascular supply; the thoracodorsal artery and vein serve as the dominant vascular pedicle and enter the muscle near its insertion. Survival of the entire muscle based solely on this dominant vascular pedicle has been documented.

1. The muscle is approached through a curvilinear incision beginning at the axilla and extending dorsally and caudally to the level of the muscle's origin (Figure 11.17)
2. Skin, subcutaneous tissue and cutaneous trunci muscle are elevated
3. The latissimus dorsi muscle is transected along its fascial origin caudally and dorsally
4. Elevation of the muscle reveals several segmental vascular branches extending from the intercostal vessels. These vessels are either cauterized or ligated and transected, allowing continued dissection of the muscle toward its origin
5. The dominant thoracodorsal artery and vein are easily seen as they course along the deep surface of the muscle
6. After identification and protection of the vascular pedicle, the tendinous insertion of the latissimus dorsi muscle is transected. The vascular pedicle is skeletonized along its length in preparation for transfer.

The size of the thoracodorsal pedicle in the cat is less than 0.8 mm; therefore, dissection of the vascular pedicle to the level of the subscapular artery and vein is recommended in this species.

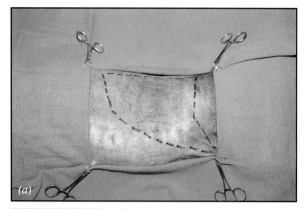

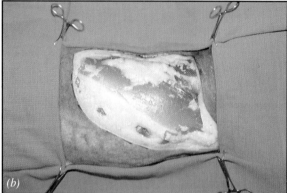

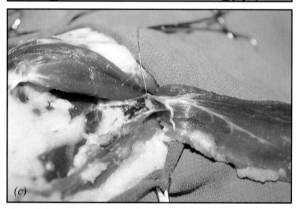

Figure 11.17: *(a) Landmarks for dissection of the latissimus dorsi muscle flap. The ventral line indicates the proposed skin incision. (b) Elevation of the skin reveals the superficial aspect of the latissimus dorsi muscle. (c) The muscle is dissected from its origin towards its insertion. Several segmental intercostal vessels must be ligated and transected near the muscle's origin. The thoracodorsal vascular pedicle is shown on the deep surface of the muscle near its insertion.*

Vascularized bone grafts

The indications, contraindications and clinical utility of non-vascularized cortical allografts are well established. They provide immediate structural integrity in instances of segmental bone loss. Ultimate success of non-vascularized allografts, however, is dependent upon revascularization followed by a process of graft resorption and new bone production that requires years. The risk of infection, delayed union, implant loosening or graft collapse is substantial.

Vascularized autogenous cortical bone grafts are immediately revascularized following transfer, and have the advantage of providing viable cellular elements that contribute actively to bone healing. They are more resistant to infection and heal more rapidly than do non-vascularized cortical allografts. After transfer, vascularized grafts rapidly remodel and hypertrophy, according to the stresses placed upon them at the recipient site. They have the disadvantage of necessitating the harvesting of a segment of cortical bone from a donor site, with an attendant risk of morbidity. Experience using microvascular transfer of cortical bone is limited in veterinary medicine, and few experimental studies exist. However, several potentially useful vascularized bone grafts have been described.

Vascularized fibula graft

The canine fibula has been used as an experimental model for the study of the biology of vascularized bone grafts:

- The fibula graft is based on either the caudal tibial or the popliteal vascular pedicle
- The popliteal artery branches into a larger cranial tibial and a smaller caudal tibial artery. The caudal tibial artery continues deep to the flexor hallicus longus muscle within the interosseous space
- The nutrient artery of the fibula arises from the caudal tibial artery, entering the fibula medially in its proximal third
- Dissection of the vascularized fibula graft, as with all vascularized bone grafts, is performed to include a surrounding myoperiosteal cuff of tissue. The flexor hallicus longus muscle belly is preserved with the graft, ensuring the integrity of the caudal tibial artery and vein.

Transfer of the fibula with the caudal tibial artery and vein results in a relatively short vascular pedicle of limited diameter. Dissection to the level of the popliteal artery and vein yields a more substantial vascular pedicle, but necessitates ligation of the cranial tibial artery and vein. Iatrogenic damage to the peroneal nerve must be avoided during proximal dissection.

Microvascular free transfer of the fibula is probably of limited use in the dog. The fibula has a small diameter and would provide little of the structural integrity needed for long bone reconstruction. However, the fibula may prove useful for augmentation of more traditional fracture repairs, or for the management of non-union fractures.

Vascularized rib graft

Microvascular transfer of the canine rib has been reported experimentally. Like the fibula, the rib is likely to be of minimal benefit to the veterinary surgeon performing reconstructive surgery, due to its curved shape and poor structural integrity. The rib is harvested with the intercostal artery and vein.

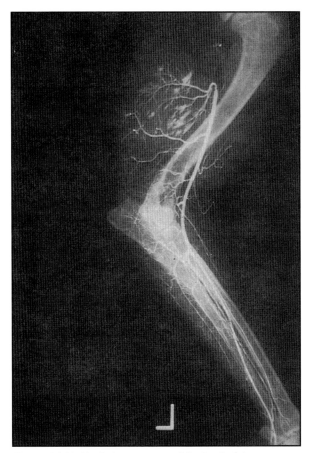

Figure 11.18: Perfusion patterns of the forelimb in a specimen after injection of barium into the brachial artery. The ulna derives its vascular supply from the caudal interosseous artery, which arises from the short common interosseous artery and extends distally in the interosseous space between the radius and the ulna.

The pedicle may be formed by either the dorsal intercostal artery and vein or the ventral intercostal artery and vein. Dorsal dissection includes the nutrient artery and vein, while ventral dissection yields a graft solely dependent upon its myoperiosteal vascular supply for survival.

Vascularized ulna graft

The canine ulna is of little importance for structural weight-bearing, and may be partially resected with few functional sequelae. Given this fact, and the innate structural properties of the ulnar diaphysis, it is a logical choice for microvascular transfer.

The ulna derives its blood supply from the caudal interosseous artery and vein (Figure 11.18). The common interosseous artery arises from the median artery at the level of the proximal radius. After entering the interosseous space from the medial side, the common interosseous artery bifurcates into caudal and cranial interosseous branches. The cranial interosseous artery emerges from the interosseous space laterally and gives rise to muscular branches to the extensor carpi ulnaris and the lateral and common digital extensor muscles. The caudal interosseous

vessels continue distally in the interosseous space, and give rise to the nutrient arteries of the radius and the ulna at the junctions of their proximal and middle thirds. Multiple periosteal branches arise throughout its course.

Vascularized ulnar transfers based on either a proximal or distal dissection have been described in dogs:

- The ulna is harvested through a caudolateral curvilinear skin incision for both proximal and distal dissections
- Fasciotomy is performed on both the extensor and flexor muscle groups to facilitate their elevation and retraction.

The proximal ulnar graft is based on the common interosseous vascular pedicle. Retraction of the extensor carpi ulnaris and lateral digital extensor muscles proximally reveals their muscular branches. These muscular branches serve as a landmark for the level of the common interosseous pedicle.

Harvesting of the proximal ulnar graft proceeds in a stepwise fashion (Figure 11.19):

1. Lateral radial periosteum is incised along the cranial surface of the abductor pollicis longus muscle, and subperiosteal dissection of the radius is continued into the interosseous space
2. The medial radial periosteum is similarly incised and elevated
3. The appropriate length of bone graft is determined, according to the requirements of the recipient site. The location of the proximal osteotomy is determined immediately proximal to the common interosseous pedicle, and the locaton of the distal osteotomy is calculated based on measurement from this point
4. Distal osteotomy is performed first and the caudal interosseous vessels are located, ligated and divided within the interosseous space
5. Circumferential subperiosteal elevation of the ulna is performed at the level of the proximal osteotomy prior to its performance
6. After completion of both osteotomies, subperiosteal elevation of the radius is continued in the interosseous space. Sharp transection of the interosseous ligament is required
7. The common interosseous artery and vein are identified and dissected to their point of origin from the median artery and vein, after elevation of the ulna.

Dissection of the distal ulna graft is similar, but is based on the caudal interosseous vascular pedicle rather than the common interosseous vessels (Figure 11.20):

1. The caudal interosseous vessels are identified, ligated and transected as they exit the interosseous space distally and caudally

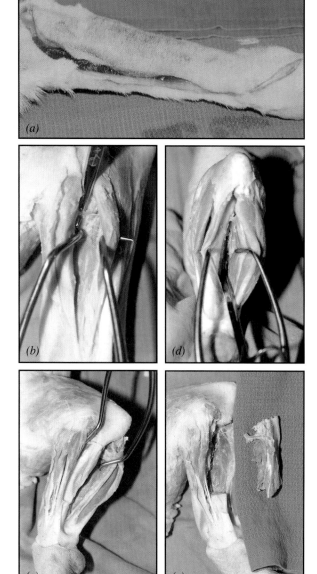

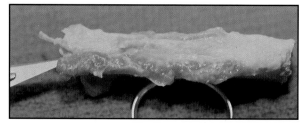

Figure 11.20: The distal ulna is dissected using the same approach as described for the proximal ulna. Proximal osteotomy is situated distal to the common interosseous vessels. The caudal interosseous vessels form the vascular pedicle.

Figure 11.19: Dissection of the proximal ulna in preparation for vascularized bone transfer. (a) An arcuate skin incision is made over the caudolateral aspect of the forelimb. (b) Fasciotomy of extensor and flexor muscle groups facilitates their elevation. Vascular branches to the extensor muscles are identified laterally and mark the level of the medially located common interosseous vessels. (c) Medial dissection of the ulna is carried into the interosseous space, taking care to preserve a myoperiosteal soft tissue cuff surrounding the bone. (d) Distal and proximal osteotomies are performed. The proximal osteotomy is situated several millimetres proximal to the level of the common interosseous vessels. The level of distal osteotomy is dependent upon the length of bone required for the reconstructive application. (e) Dissection of the specimen has been completed. The short common interosseous vascular pedicle is shown.

2. The ulna is circumferentially dissected and osteotomized immediately distal to this level
3. Incision and elevation of the medial and lateral radial periosteum is performed as described for the proximal ulna graft

4. Proximal osteotomy of the ulna is performed at a level that will yield 2–3 cm greater length than is required at the recipient site. The ulna is carefully dissected subperiosteally at this level to avoid trauma to the interosseous vessels, and proximal osteotomy is performed
5. The ulna is carefully elevated and the caudal interosseous artery and vein are ligated and transected
6. The caudal interosseous artery and vein are subsequently dissected under the operating microscope for a length of 2–3 cm from the proximal osteotomy, and the 'extra' length of ulna is excised to provide the length needed for reconstruction.

Both proximal and distal ulnar grafts are harvested with a myoperiosteal sleeve, including the ulnar head of the deep digital flexor, the pronator quadratus and the abductor pollicis longus muscles. The nutrient artery of the ulna is incorporated in the proximal dissection, while distal dissection results in preservation of the myoperiosteal blood supply only. Both result in predictable survival. Proximal dissection has the disadvantage of requiring osteotomy of the ulna near the elbow joint.

Fixation of vascularized grafts at the recipient site deserves special mention. Since vascularized grafts depend substantially or wholly upon the integrity of their myoperiosteal blood supply, it is imperative that fixation techniques be used that minimize embarrassment of this vasculature. Therefore, external skeletal fixation is recommended (Figure 11.21).

Compound flaps

Compound flaps refer to flaps that incorporate more than one type of tissue: musculocutaneous flaps, osteocutaneous flaps and myo-osseous flaps are examples.

As with all microvascular flaps, the only prerequisite is that all the tissues are nourished by a single source artery and vein. A detailed knowledge of vascular anatomy allows a great deal of flexibility in flap design.

The trapezius flap may be harvested as a myocutaneous flap by preserving the direct cutaneous branch of the superficial cervical artery and vein. The associated axial pattern skin flap is then included with dissection of the trapezius muscle. Skin is either used to resurface the muscle, or is dissected free of the underlying muscle to resurface portions of the wound bed adjacent to the muscle flap (Figure 11.22).

The latissimus dorsi flap may be harvested as a myocutaneous flap by inclusion of the direct cutaneous vessels arising from the thoracodorsal artery and vein. The thoracodorsal axial pattern skin flap is then used in a manner similar to that described for the trapezius myocutaneous flap. Skin directly overlying the latissimus dorsi muscle can also be included as a myocutaneous flap without preservation of the direct cutaneous artery of the thoracodorsal skin flap. This region of skin is supplied by intercostal cutaneous perforators and does not mandate inclusion of the direct cutaneous artery and vein in the flap design.

The scapular spine has been successfully included with the trapezius flap, resulting in the formation of a myo-osseous or osteomusculocutaneous flap (Figure 11.23). The scapular spine does not lie within the primary angiosome of the superficial cervical vessels, but survives based on blood flow through 'choke vessels'. These are small calibre vascular channels that

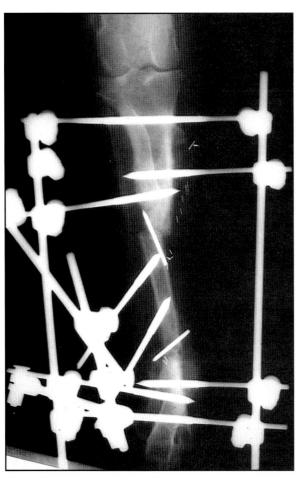

Figure 11.21: *External skeletal fixation is recommended for stabilization of vascularized bone transfers. This form of fixation minimizes injury to periosteal vasculature.*

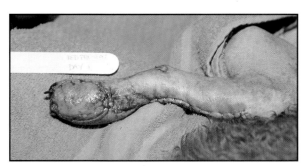

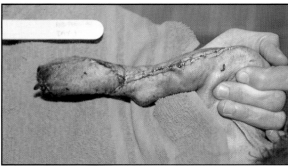

Figure 11.22: *Composite flaps can be used to facilitate reconstruction of large wounds. The muscular portion of a trapezius myocutaneous flap has been used to reconstruct the lateral and dorsal aspects of this wound, while the cutaneous portion has been used for resurfacing the medial aspect of the wound.*

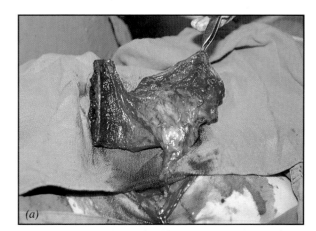

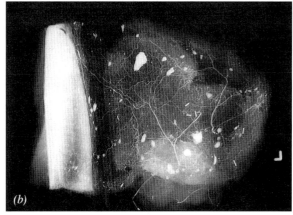

Figure 11.23: *(a) A dissected trapezius myo-osseous flap. The flap consists of the trapezius muscle and the scapular spine. (b) The scapular spine does not lie within the primary angiosome of the prescapular branch of the superficial cervical artery and vein. Survival of the scapular portion of this flap is dependent upon vascular flow through small 'choke' vessels that interconnect adjacent angiosomes.*

connect adjacent angiosomes. In the event of vascular injury, choke vessels increase in size, allowing a redistribution of blood supply. The trapezius–scapular spine myo-osseous flap may be used for the reconstruction of small bone defects (such as metatarsal or metacarpal injuries) associated with extensive soft tissue trauma.

REFERENCES AND FURTHER READING

Basher AWP, Fowler FD, Bowen CV, Clark EG and Crosby NL (1990) Microneurovascular free digital pad transfer in the dog. *Veterinary Surgery* **19(3)**, 226–231

Brown K, Marie P, Lyszakowski T, Daniel R and Cruess R (1983) Epiphysial growth after free fibular transfer with and without microvascular anastomosis. *Journal of Bone and Joint Surgery (Br)* **65B(4)**, 493–501

Degner DA, Walshaw R, Lanz O, Rosenstein D and Smith RJ (1996) The medial saphenous fasciocutaneous free flap in dogs. *Veterinary Surgery* **25(2)**, 105–113

Fisher J and Wood MB (1987) Experimental comparison of bone revascularization by musculocutaneous and cutaneous free flaps. *Plastic Reconstructive Surgery* **79**, 81–90

Fowler JD, Miller CW, Bowen V and Johnston GH (1987) Transfer of free vascular cutaneous flaps by microvascular anastomosis: result in six dogs. *Veterinary Surgery* **16(6)**, 446–450

Levitt L, Fowler JD, Longley M, Bowen V and Wilkinson AA (1988) A developmental model for free vascularized bone transfers in the dog. *Veterinary Surgery* **17(4)**, 194–202

Miller CW, Chang P and Bowen V (1986) Identification and transfer of free cutaneous flaps by microvascular anastomosis in the dog. *Veterinary Surgery* **15(2)**, 199–204

Moens NMM and Fowler JD (1997) The microvascular carpal foot pad flap: vascular anatomy and surgical technique. *Veterinary Compendium of Orthopedic Traumatology* **10**, 183–186

Nicoll SA, Fowler JD, Remedios AM, Clapson JB and George D (1996) Development of a free latissimus dorsi muscle flap in cats. *Veterinary Surgery* **25(1)**, 40–48

Ostrup LT and Fredrickson JM (1974) Distant transfer of a free, living bone graft by microvascular anastomoses. *Plastic Reconstructive Surgery* **54(3)**, 274–285

Philibert D and Fowler JD (1993) The trapezius osteomusculocutaneous flap in dogs. *Veterinary Surgery* **22(6)**, 444–450

Philibert D, Fowler JD and Clapson JB (1992) Free microvascular transplantation of the trapezius musculocutaneous flap in dogs. *Veterinary Surgery* **21(6)**, 435–440

Szentimrey D and Fowler D (1994) The anatomic basis of a free vascularized bone graft based on the canine distal ulna. *Veterinary Surgery* **23(6)**, 529–533

CHAPTER TWELVE

Special Considerations in Wound Management

John M. Williams

CHRONIC DRAINING SINUSES

A sinus is a fibrous tissue tract lined by chronic, oedematous, granulating tissue and is usually associated with purulent, serous or serosanguinous discharge. A fistula differs from a sinus tract in that it connects the skin surface with a mucosal surface of a viscus and may be lined with epithelium.

Causes of sinus tracts include bacterial infection, foreign bodies deep within tissues, bone sequestra, surgical implants (sutures, meshes, orthopaedic implants) and neoplasia. The clinical signs associated with sinus tracts (pain, swelling, discharge) may be ameliorated and can subside completely when treated with courses of antibiotics. However, the tract and clinical signs will recur after the medication is stopped. All sinus tracts should therefore be thoroughly investigated and explored surgically to determine and eliminate (if possible) the cause. If the cause is not eliminated, a tract will recur. Chronic sinus tracts can be extremely frustrating to manage for the patient, client and veterinary surgeon, as small fragments of foreign material can be elusive and repeated surgical intervention may be required.

It is important to develop a systematic approach to the investigation of sinus tracts. This should include:

- A thorough history, e.g. working gundogs may be more prone to foreign body penetration from working in thick undergrowth
- Thorough clinical examination, looking for evidence of concurrent disease, especially if neoplasia is suspected
- Palpation and probing of the tract, with the patient under general anaesthesia, to determine its likely extent
- Plain/survey radiographs of the area (Figure 12.1). It may be necessary to radiograph some way from the exit site as some tracts can extend considerable distances. Plain radiographs may reveal radiodense foreign bodies, bone sequestra, areas of discospondylitis, or surgical swabs (sponges) inadvertently left following some previous surgery
- Instillation of radiopaque contrast material (fistulogram) to delineate the extent of the tract should be considered. Fistulography can be useful in some cases where it may allow delineation of a foreign body (filling defect in the tract) and the full extent of the tract to be shown. It can be frustrating in some cases as contrast does not always remain in the tract and may leak out of the tract (Figure 12.2), especially if injected under pressure. If the tract is wide enough a Foley catheter is inserted and the bulb

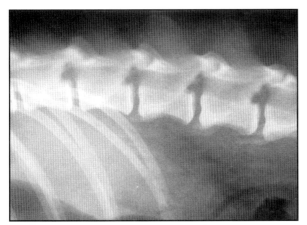

Figure 12.1: Plain lateral abdominal radiograph of an English Springer Spaniel that had a discharging sinus on the left flank. At surgery, the sinus was found to extend to the intervertebral space between thoracic vertebrae 11 and 12. Nocardia *was cultured from the disk space.*

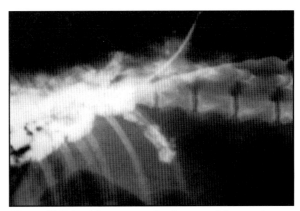

Figure 12.2: Positive contrast fistulogram of the case in Figure 12.1. Note the delineation of the tract and the loss of contrast medium from the sinus. The contrast medium did not enter the whole length of the tract.

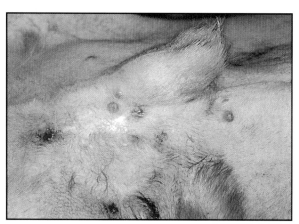

Figure 12.3: *Multiple sinus tracts, visible following hair clipping.*

gently inflated (to prevent leakage); for narrow tracts a 16- or 18-gauge intravenous catheter can be used. Sterile iodine-based water-soluble contrast is injected slowly. It is helpful even when a Foley catheter is used to apply some digital pressure to the proximal tract to reduce the occurrence of backflow
- A dye such as methylene blue can be instilled into the tract to facilitate surgical exploration
- Prior to surgery, clip and aseptically prepare a large area around the tract, especially if the extent of the tract is unknown (Figure 12.3)
- Explore and excise all tracts encountered
- If foreign material is found look for more! There is nothing more frustrating than a patient re-presenting some weeks or months later due to recurrence of a problem that was thought to have been solved
- All previously implanted surgical materials should be removed
- If no foreign material is found, dissect out the tract and close the wound. Submit the tract for bacteriological culture and sensitivity as well as for histopathology.

PHARYNGEAL STICK PENETRATION INJURIES

Injuries to the canine pharynx are infrequent, but the pharynx is particularly susceptible to wooden stick injury, particularly in those breeds which chase or carry sticks. Such injuries have been most commonly described in young, medium to large dogs, especially Collie types. This has been suggested to be due to the 'head down' position that larger dogs adopt when picking up sticks from the ground (White and Lane, 1988).

Pharyngeal stick injuries present either acutely, within a short time of the injury occurring, or chronically, when they may present only with a discharging sinus (see above).

Acutely presenting patients will either have a known history of stick injury or, if presented within a few days of trauma, they usually have dysphagia. This is due either to temporomasseteric trauma or to pharyngeal laceration and secondary cellulitis. Pharyngocervical pain is common. The potential track

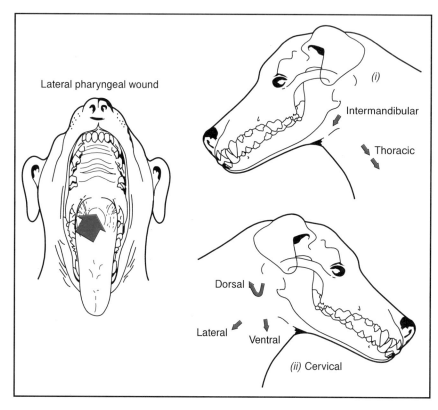

Figure 12.4: *Potential paths of a lateral pharyngeal stick injury: (i) penetrating the intermandibular or cranial thoracic region; (ii) entering the cervical parapharyngeal tissues.*

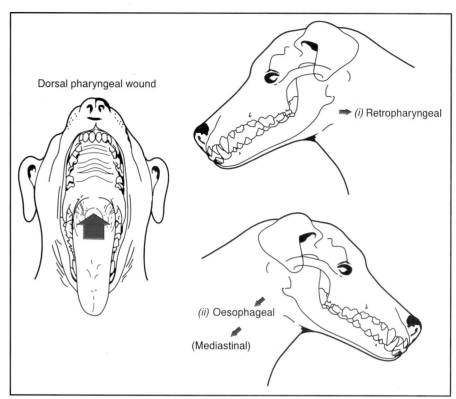

Dorsal pharyngeal wound

(i) Retropharyngeal

(ii) Oesophageal

(Mediastinal)

Figure 12.5: Potential paths of a dorsal pharyngeal stick injury. Sticks entering the mouth from directly in front of the dog may (i) enter steeply, lacerating the soft palate and entering the retropharynx, or (ii) enter at a lower angle and be more likely to penetrate the oesophagus.

taken by a stick entering the oropharynx has been well described (White and Lane, 1988) and two common routes are shown (Figures 12.4 and 12.5). Crepitation due to subcutaneous air accumulation may be noted within a few days, occurring secondary to pharyngeal or oesophageal lacerations.

The fresh pharyngeal or suspected pharyngeal laceration should be explored immediately, in order to minimize the development of chronic complications. This is especially important if oesophageal penetration has occurred. In the author's experience oesophageal lacerations should be explored within 24 hours of trauma, otherwise wound dehiscence is common with subsequent death of the patient. Prior to obtaining results of culture and sensitivity from the wound (swab and tissue culture should be done); broad-spectrum intravenous antibiotics should be instituted, with the addition of metronidazole to combat anaerobic infection. For all suspected dorsal or lateral pharyngeal penetration injuries, a ventral midline cervical approach should be used. This will allow the full extent of the injury to be established and the area to be explored fully for fragments of foreign body.

Pharyngeal and oesophageal lacerations should be debrided and sutured with 1.5 or 2 metric absorbable material (the oesophagus is best closed with two layers of simple interrupted sutures). The oesophageal wound should be supported, either by suturing the cranial portion of the sternothyroid muscle to the wound or with lengthened omentum (see below). A gastrostomy tube should be placed (see below) for 7 days to allow healing to occur. Drains should be placed in the area of the dissection (see Figure 2.10).

Where the stick has penetrated the retrobulbar area, drainage is achieved via the oral cavity by using a haemostat to enlarge the wound or by penetrating the pharyngeal mucosa caudal to the last molar.

DERMOID CYST/PILONIDAL SINUS

This is an inherited condition of Rhodesian Ridgebacks (which has also been reported in Boxers and Shih-Tzus). There is a failure of the neural tube to separate completely from the skin in the embryo. The extent of failure is variable but the defect may reach from the skin to the dura mater.

Diagnosis is usually made based on the breed and age at presentation. These are usually young dogs with palpable cords of tissue in the dorsal cervical area cranial to the characteristic 'ridge' along the dorsum. Other tracts can develop in the region secondary to the deep pyoderma which may occur. Occasionally dogs may exhibit neurological signs if the tract extends to the dura mater and a concurrent meningiomyelitis occurs. The full extent of the tract should be defined by performing a fistulogram using a non-ionic iodine-based water-soluble contrast medium (Figure 12.6). If there is communication with the spinal cord a cervical myelogram may also be of value.

In order to resolve the problem, surgical excision of the epithelium-lined tract is required. A dorsal approach to the neck is employed and the surgeon must be prepared for a deep dissection through the neck muscles. In the majority of cases the tracts narrow at, or just dorsal to, the nuchal ligament. Occasionally it is necessary to

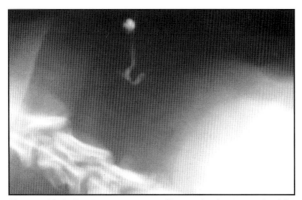

Figure 12.6: Positive contrast radiograph of a 4-month-old Rhodesian Ridgeback, showing the extent of the pilonidal sinus.

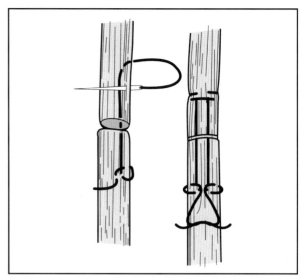

Figure 12.7: A modified Kessler locking loop suture pattern for reapposing cut tendons.

split the nuchal ligament; if this is done, then on closure the ligament should be reapposed with a modified Kessler locking loop suture pattern (Figure 12.7) using non-absorbable suture material such as polypropylene.

A proportion of these tracts stop immediately dorsal to a vertebral spinous process, the dorsal portion of which should be excised with the tract. If the tract extends into the dura mater, a dorsal laminectomy is required and the part of the dura connecting with the sinus is excised with it. Samples of tract should be submitted for both bacterial culture and histopathology. Postoperative seroma formation is common at this site and drainage must be established; closed suction drainage is preferable (see Chapter 6).

The prognosis is good for cases with no evidence of meningiomyelitis, but if this is present then the prognosis is guarded. Though the heritability of this condition is not fully understood, owners should be advised not to breed from affected animals.

ANAL FURUNCULOSIS

Anal furunculosis (perianal fistulation) is a frustrating disease encountered commonly in German Shepherd Dogs and Border Collies, and is characterized by chronic infection and ulceration of the tissues around the anus (Figure 12.8). More importantly, there are often deeply infiltrating sinus tracts which can form true fistulae with the rectum.

The underlying cause of this disease remains elusive. Recent studies have shown that dogs respond well to immunosuppressive drugs (Mathews *et al.*, 1997), which suggests an immune-mediated component. There is also some evidence that there is an association with inflammatory bowel disease as there is in humans who suffer from Crohn's disease and concurrent perianal fistulae (Harkin *et al.*, 1996; Mathews *et al.*, 1997). Factors that have been proposed as perpetuating the problem include the conformation of the German Shepherd Dog, allowing the broad base of the tail to remain in close contact

with the anus and spreading a thin film of faeces over the perineal region. Anal sacculitis is also a perpetuating factor; the anal sacs should be removed if surgery is likely to be successful.

The range of clinical signs seen with anal furunculosis varies immensely, from the case which shows few signs, apart from licking the perianal region, to the

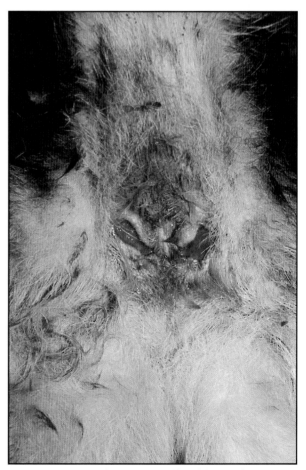

Figure 12.8: Typical appearance of anal furunculosis.

advanced case where damage and scarring of the anal sphincter and rectum prevents normal dilation of the anus. These dogs can show severe faecal tenesmus, dyschezia and pain. Conversely, some dogs with severe anal furunculosis lose the ability to close the anal sphincter and become faecally incontinent.

No single technique has been shown to result consistently in a cure for anal furunculosis. The author currently favours open excision of the anal sacs, combined with sharp dissection of the sinuses, closure of the dead space with fine synthetic absorbable sutures, and primary wound closure. Surgical removal of the infected tissue, with or without reconstruction of the surrounding skin, provides a reasonable outcome in a majority of cases.

Surgery is carried out with the patient placed in sternal recumbency with the tail tied upward and forward and the hindlimbs hanging over the end of the table. To facilitate surgery, the table can be tipped at an angle to raise the animal's tail end, taking care not to exceed 25–30 degrees. A tilt greater than this may compromise respiration, due to cranial shift of the abdominal organs. The area is clipped and prepared as aseptically as possible. Enemas are avoided to prevent perianal leakage of liquid faeces, gauze swabs soaked in 1% povidone–iodine may be inserted per rectum and the perineal area is draped out.

The procedure of choice for removing the anal sacs is open excision. Resins and other materials to pack the anal sac are to be avoided, as they may leak into surrounding tissues producing a chronic focus for infection.

Anal sacculectomy is a straightforward procedure requiring no specialized instrumentation.

1. A small haemostat or scalpel guide is inserted through the anal sac opening and incised on to with a No. 15 scalpel blade (Figure 12.9). With this technique there is minimal risk of damaging the deep portion of the anal sphincter muscle or the caudal rectal branch of the pudendal nerve
2. Using fine thumb forceps, the anal sac lining is grasped and dissected free from the surrounding tissues (Figure 12.10). In severe disease it is common to find only remnants of the anal sacs, which must be removed
3. Sharp excision of all sinuses and tracts is carried out, paying careful attention to haemostasis.

It may be necessary in severe cases to excise part or all of the external anal sphincter muscle. Owners should be warned of this possibility with its attendant potential risk of postoperative faecal incontinence.

Postoperative care should include suitable analgesia with either an opioid or a non-steroidal anti-inflammatory drug such as carprofen. The intraoperative use of epidural analgesia can be invaluable in the immediate postoperative period. Wound interference may be a problem and an Elizabethan collar may help. If wound

dehiscence occurs, and is not excessive, it can be allowed to heal by secondary intention. All cases should be checked 2–3 days after surgery.

Recurrence is not uncommon and all cases should be reassessed after 6 weeks when further surgery may be contemplated. A proportion of dogs do not respond to surgery.

Due to the possible link with inflammatory bowel conditions, the use of immunosuppressive agents has been reported. Two distinct treatment regimens have been described. One regimen used moderate doses of prednisolone, initially at 2 mg/kg for 2 weeks then reducing the dose over 4–6 weeks (Harkin *et al.*, 1996). The other used cyclosporin, a potent immunosuppressive agent that requires monitoring of blood levels on a weekly basis to ensure that therapeutic levels are maintained (Mathews *et al.*, 1997). Results from these two studies, so far, suggest that such regimens should be considered as part of the future management of anal furunculosis/perianal fistulae.

Interestingly, in human patients perianal fistulation is frequently managed successfully by application of topical hydroactive dressings (see Chapter 5) for several weeks. This is not a practical alternative for most dogs!

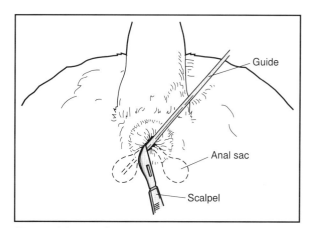

Figure 12.9: A guide is inserted through the anal sac opening and incised on to with a No. 15 scalpel blade.

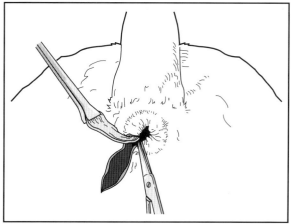

Figure 12.10: The anal sac is grasped and dissected free.

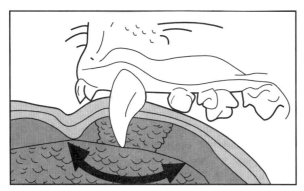

Figure 12.11: A cat's canine teeth can cause wounds to tissues underlying the skin wound.

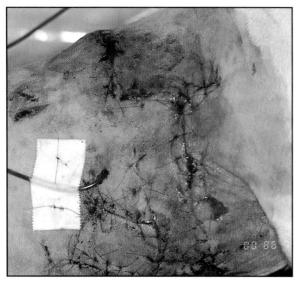

Figure 12.12: The thorax of a Jack Russell Terrier, 5 days post trauma. The dog had been bitten on the thorax, resulting in fractured ribs, an open pneumothorax and extensive skin loss. The wounds were treated as open wounds following aggressive debridement of devitalized tissues.

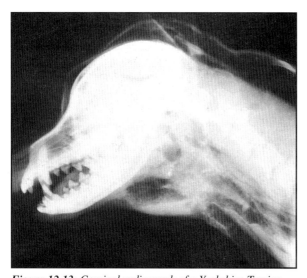

Figure 12.13: Cervical radiograph of a Yorkshire Terrier that had been bitten on the neck 24 hours previously. Note the extensive subcutaneous emphysema. Careful re-evaluation of the original radiograph revealed damage to the tracheal rings.

BITE WOUNDS

The mouths of both dogs and cats are heavily contaminated with aerobic, anaerobic, Gram-positive and Gram-negative bacteria. Cats, in particular, have abundant numbers of *Pasteurella multocida*, a frequent cause of cellulitis. All bite wounds are contaminated and must be managed as such. In addition to inoculating bacteria under the skin, the jaws and teeth of animals can cause severe trauma, not only to the skin but especially to the underlying deep tissues (Figure 12.11). The jaws of large dogs in particular produce significant tearing and crushing forces, within the deeper tissue, which makes smaller dogs and cats very susceptible to injury. Common sites of injury are the neck, thorax and abdomen, where there is potential for damage to the airway, oesophagus, thoracic cage and intra-abdominal organs, notably the kidneys. Such damage also leads to devitalization of underlying tissues, which will then make an ideal substrate for bacterial colonization.

It is essential that *all* suspected bite wounds are examined carefully and not dismissed as trivial puncture marks on the skin. What is seen at the initial presentation is usually just the 'tip of the iceberg' with respect to damage to the underlying structures. It is also of paramount importance to assess the patient as a whole, because if there is trauma to the upper airway, oesophagus or thorax this will need dealing with promptly.

Dogs and cats with suspected bite wounds should be clipped over the area so as to note the full extent of any contusions and to find small puncture wounds, which can be readily masked by hair. All bite wounds should be explored surgically and debrided (Figure 12.12); prior to doing this it may be necessary to stabilize the patient. If there is severe neck trauma with transection of the trachea, immediate surgical intervention may be required in order to establish a patent airway. If wounds are not explored such a patient will frequently be re-presented in 24–48 hours with complications associated with the deep tissue trauma (Figure 12.13).

BURNS

Burn injuries have the potential to destroy large areas of skin which can result in the loss of two of its most important functions: prevention of loss of body fluids; and protection against infection.

The severity of the clinical signs seen depends on both the surface area involved and the depth of skin loss. Fortunately, burns are not a common presentation in small animal practice, with only sporadic reports in the literature. In comparison, human burn injuries account for some 10,000 hospital admissions in the UK and an estimated 115,000 hospital admissions in the USA annually. Causes of burns in animals include: exposure to fire and smoke; accidental or malicious application of hot liquids; electricity; chemicals; and the effects of radiation (both ultraviolet and X-ray). Iatrogenic burns are the commonest in small animals, due to hot air dryers, electric and water-heated pads, and poorly earthed diathermy units.

In order to manage a burn patient successfully the clinician must identify the severity and extent of the skin trauma. This allows measures to be instituted which will combat the problems encountered following severe fluid loss and infection. In addition to skin lesions, many burn patients may also have airway damage, due either to smoke inhalation or to direct thermal injury to oropharyngeal and airway tissues. Clearly such injuries must be attended to without delay.

Following thermal skin injury, patients suffer 'burn shock', a series of severe pathophysiological changes which are secondary to capillary fluid and protein loss and are complicated by sepsis and immunocompromise. The majority of our understanding of burn injury is extrapolated from human burn patients. This can serve us well in the basic understanding of the disease mechanisms involved but it is important to remember that dogs and cats have a substantial hair coat and that the microanatomy of their skin differs substantially from that of humans.

Understanding the underlying pathophysiology of the burn patient together with basic wound healing

allows us to develop strategies for patient management. To understand the burn victim fully, it is easier to consider systems in isolation, though when dealing with a patient we deal with the problems as a whole.

Pathophysiology of burns

Skin injury

The area and depth of skin damage are the most important factors in determining the extent of pathophysiological change in the patient. This damage is a function of the temperature reached and the duration of contact with the skin (Figure 12.14); cellular death begins at 40°C. Burns are classified as *superficial partial, deep partial* and *full thickness* skin loss (Figure 12.15). This classification is important with respect to the subsequent healing of the burn wound.

Superficial partial thickness skin loss: Hair follicles and a substantial part of the dermis are spared. This is the least serious of the skin injuries inflicted by burns and is recognized less often in cats and dogs than in people due to the insulating properties of the hair coat. As there is no superficial vascular plexus as found in humans, the degree of erythema is less and blisters rarely form. This is the type of burn suffered following exposure to ultraviolet radiation or following therapeutic doses of irradiation. It produces moderate erythema, followed by desquamation and thickening of the skin. As the injury is very superficial there are minimal systemic effects and the skin heals rapidly by re-epithelialization.

Deep partial thickness skin loss: Leaves only a small number of hair follicles and part of the dermis following a burn. Such thermal trauma produces a marked inflammatory response. Subdermal oedema due to increased vascular permeability follows activation of the complement system, the creation of free oxygen radicals and xanthine oxidase products. Though burn depth can be difficult to assess at the time of injury, such wounds are classically described as being moist, blanching on pressure and responding to pain stimuli. A deep partial thickness skin wound may heal by

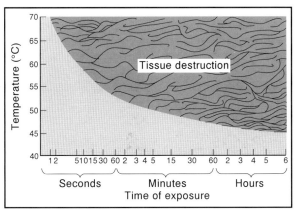

Figure 12.14: Tissue damage from burning depends on temperature and time of exposure.

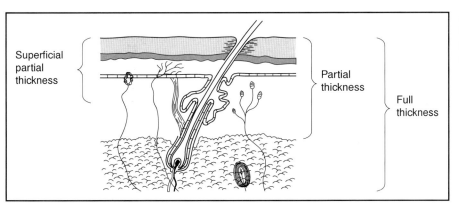

Figure 12.15: Schematic representation of the depth of skin damage caused by a burn injury.

second intention but this tends to be slow due to a paucity of epithelial elements. It is essential that such a wound is managed correctly (see below) or it may transform to full thickness skin loss.

Full thickness skin loss: No dermis or epidermal remnants survive and there is often thermal injury to deeper structures. There is severe inflammation and oedema and systemic signs are common. This type of burn therefore carries a much poorer prognosis.

Area affected

The amount of body surface area affected has a marked influence on the severity of systemic effects. The most important early pathological change is that of increased capillary permeability. The extent of capillary damage is closely related to the percentage total body surface area (TBSA) burned. To assess TBSA we can adapt and apply the useful '*Rule of Nine*' which is used for adult human burns (Figure 12.16). There will be breed and age variation to this 'rule', but it does allow a rapid evaluation for the management of the patient. For any canine or feline patient with full or partial thickness burns of more than 50% TBSA, euthanasia may be advisable due to the severity of the injuries, though dogs and cats may survive with such injuries (see Chapter 2).

Airway injury

Any animal who suffers burns around the head will develop severe oropharyngeal oedema, especially if the thermal agent has affected the inside of the oropharynx or the upper respiratory tract. Stridor and respiratory distress develop within hours of a serious thermal injury, and patients will require either emergency intubation or, more likely, emergency tracheostomy tube placement. It is fortunately rare for thermal injuries to extend into the lower respiratory tract, due to the extremely efficient heat dissipation ability of the upper airway. When thermal injury of the lower respiratory tract does occur, the animal will experience bronchospasm, presenting with productive, wheezing coughs.

In addition to oedema secondary to burns, patients are also susceptible to carbon monoxide poisoning and smoke inhalation. Incomplete combustion of materials frequently leads to carbon monoxide production, which may be as high as 8% in inhaled air in house fires. Since carbon monoxide has a much higher affinity for haemoglobin than does oxygen, levels as low as 1% CO in inhaled air may produce carboxyhaemoglobin levels of >50% within 10 minutes. Generally, levels above 60% are associated with a high mortality rate. Clinically, such patients will have cherry red mucosae. In the absence of a hyperbaric oxygen chamber, oxygen supplied by mask or via a tracheostomy tube will help reduce the half-life of carboxyhaemoglobin to 45–60 minutes.

Smoke inhalation injuries, though uncommon, occur due to the toxic material found in smoke particles, which are directly irritant to the tracheobronchial tree and produce mucosal inflammation, oedema and necrosis plus pulmonary oedema. In some cases tracheal mucosal sloughing is so severe that the debris may physically obstruct the lower airways. This may also be associated with the development of pulmonary oedema, usually within 72

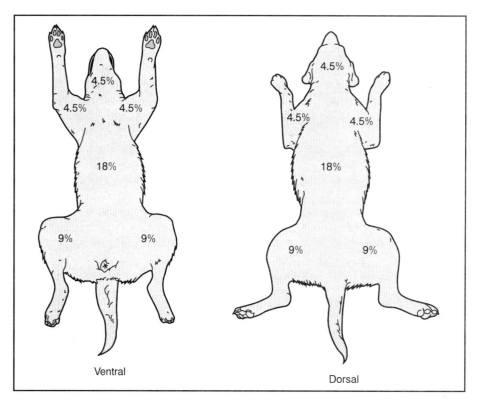

Figure 12.16: The '*Rule of Nine*', adapted from human medicine. A rapid and effective estimate of the percentage total body surface area affected can be calculated using this diagram.

Ventral

Dorsal

hours of the inhalational injury; its occurrence in human patients is associated with a mortality rate as high as 70%. Currently, the best option for management of smoke inhalation is the use of bronchodilators in conjunction with humidified oxygen delivered by positive pressure ventilation.

The damage to the tracheobronchial tree makes bacterial infection a common sequel and this is a major cause of death. Pneumonic infection arises either by contamination via the airway or by haematogenous spread.

Fluid loss

Following a severe burn there will be varying degrees of capillary damage. The increase in capillary permeability leads to loss of fluid, primarily into the intracellular spaces; the vast majority of this fluid loss is not seen and is therefore readily overlooked. The leakage is maximal during the first 8 hours after burning and then gradually decreases over 48–72 hours until the animal creates enough fluid to compensate. The exact timing will depend on age and degree of damage; fluid balance returns more quickly in the young animal and more slowly in those with extensive burns. With burns affecting up to 20–30% TBSA, fluid leakage tends to be local to the wound site; for burns affecting >30% TBSA, the increase in capillary permeability tends to be generalized. Even with a 20% TBSA burn, 28% of the plasma volume of a dog can be lost within 6 hours. When the affected TBSA is >40% the animal may lose up to 50% of its plasma volume within 2–3 hours.

Electrolytes

Burn patients suffer from electrolyte imbalances. Thermal injury has a profound effect on cell membrane potential; this, combined with the affinity that sodium has for denatured collagen in burn wounds, leads to a major shift of both sodium ions and water into the interstitial and intracellular spaces. Hyponatraemia rarely becomes a clinical problem as intravenous therapy is with sodium-containing fluids.

In the burn patient there may be an early transient hyperkalaemia due to erythrocyte destruction; this is rarely a problem as long as renal function is maintained. Diuresis secondary to fluid therapy may precipitate hypokalaemia requiring the addition of potassium to the fluids. Potassium can be added at 20 mEq/l and administered at a rate up to 0.5 mEq/kg/h. Any hypokalaemia will be accentuated if there is respiratory alkalosis due to hyperventilation.

Sepsis

Surface burn wounds are extremely susceptible to secondary infection. Initially the wound will be contaminated only by the skin's resident flora. By 2 weeks post burn there is colonization of the wound by exogenous bacteria, in particular:

- Haemolytic streptococci
- Haemolytic staphylococci
- *Pseudomonas aeruginosa.*

Pseudomanads pose a special problem in the burn patient as they can cause death without the animal exhibiting signs of fever or leucocytosis. The risk of developing sepsis increases with increasing TBSA affected; if the TBSA affected is less than 30% then sepsis is generally not a problem. Burn sepsis may go unnoticed until the eschar that has formed over the wound begins to separate. The eschar is the brown/black, leather-like, discoloured area which is the result of the heat damage to skin and other tissues, which eventually becomes organized as tough collagen elements.

Infection is a major contributor to mortality in burn patients and is in part due to the severe compromise to defence mechanisms, which prevents the patient mounting an effective response. There is:

- Loss of skin as external barrier
- Depletion of complement and other factors of the non-specific defence system
- Poor specific immunity due to loss of immunoglobulins (IgA and IgG) through vascular permeability and compounded by depression of cell-mediated immunity.

As a consequence, septicaemia is a common sequel to local wound infection in burn patients and must be treated aggressively with high doses of systemic antibiotics, based on the results of bacterial blood culture and sensitivity tests.

Anaemia

Anaemia is a common consequence of burns and occurs due to a number of mechanisms. There is immediate thermal destruction of red blood cells, followed by physiological lysis some hours later. In addition, some red cells are so morphologically damaged that they will be filtered out by the spleen. Erythrocyte membrane damage also occurs due to various catecholamines, prostaglandins and altered plasma lipids, and this reduces red cell life span. Patients with severe burns also have reduced levels of erythropoietin, depressing erythropoiesis and resulting in a normocytic, normochromic anaemia.

Metabolic response

Due to massive capillary leakage, a large amount of protein is lost both through the wound and into the intravascular spaces. This sets up a massive negative nitrogen balance and the body attempts to compensate with increases in both metabolic and catabolic rates to 1–1.5 times normal; this increases the patient's nutritional protein requirement by 2–3.5 times. Even with high-calorie high-nitrogen nutritional supplementation it is not possible to reverse the process until healing is complete. In order to address this, a suitable high-quality commercial diet which has the correct protein/energy balance should be used. This will at least go some way towards countering the severe negative nitrogen balance.

Managing the patient with burns

With any thermal injury it is essential to remove the source as quickly as possible and to cool the tissue rapidly with cold water or ice. Large wounds should be covered during transportation; cling film is a suitable covering which will help protect the wound. Applying a dressing to the affected area will produce some local analgesic effect.

It is essential to deal with any life-threatening problem the patient may have. Notably there is a need to check and maintain an airway and to attend to any evidence of burn shock by fluid administration.

Fluid therapy

As it is not possible to stem the leakage of fluid, it is essential to maintain the patient's circulating volume, otherwise hypovolaemic shock with the potential for renal failure will occur.

For fluid replacement:

- Lactated Ringer's (Hartmann's) solution should be used initially
- Avoid colloids during the first 24 hours after burning, as the capillaries are permeable to molecules up to a molecular weight of 125,000; therefore the colloid will be lost into the extravascular space along with the plasma.

The rate of fluid administration can be calculated based on a number of different formulae. A suitable rate for the first 24 hours post burn is that based on the Parkland Hospital Formula:

- Use 4 ml Hartmann's solution per kg per %TBSA
- Give half of the calculated fluid requirement in the first 8 hours post thermal injury
- Give the remaining half over the next 16 hours

After the first 24 hours, colloids or plasma are added to the fluid therapy regimen to maintain both cardiac output and plasma volume:

- The dose of colloid needed is 0.3–0.5 ml colloid per kg per % TBSA
- Ultimately the rate of fluid administration depends on the responses of the patient, i.e. heart rate, capillary refill time, and urine output
- The patient should produce between 1 and 1.5 ml/kg/h of urine if adequate renal perfusion is occurring; if not, then fluid administration rates should be increased.

Pain relief

It is important to provide pain relief for burn patients; opioids should be the first choice. The use of corticosteroids and non-steroidal anti-inflammatories is controversial. There is no evidence that corticosteroids will be harmful; NSAIDs are best avoided until renal function is clearly established.

Total parenteral nutrition

A burn patient may be unable to eat, particularly if it is suffering from oropharyngeal oedema. In such cases non-oral enteral feeding techniques should be considered. In the majority of cases the intestinal tract will be functioning and all that is required is a form of tube feeding which bypasses the oral cavity.

Total parenteral nutrition (TPN) should only be considered in those cases where there is intestinal dysfunction. TPN is a high-risk option in these cases due to the possibility of introducing infection in an already immunocompromised patient. Either tube oesophagostomy or tube gastrostomy will work well. Oesophagostomy placement is particularly well suited to cats and is less likely to cause problems than a pharyngostomy tube. Oesophagostomy tubes are placed with the patient anaesthetized and in right lateral recumbency, with the left cervical area clipped and prepared aseptically:

1. Long curved artery forceps are placed in the proximal oesophagus and the tip pushed towards the skin
2. A 10- to 14-gauge needle is pushed through the skin between the jaws of the forceps
3. A catheter is passed down the needle into the oesophagus. The catheter (14–18 French) should extend so that it terminates in the distal third of the oesophagus. Measure from the point of proposed oesophageal entry to the seventh intercostal space; this will minimize the risks of gastro-oesophageal reflux.

Alternatively, a gastrostomy tube can be placed. This is done either transabdominally with the aid of an endoscope (percutaneous endoscopic gastrostomy) or surgically via a paracostal incision:

1. A left-sided tube gastrostomy is performed via a sublumbar paracostal incision
2. A silicone 20- to 26-gauge Foley catheter is placed through the skin and muscles caudal to the skin incision via a tunnel created by blunt dissection with artery forceps through a stab incision in the skin
3. The Foley catheter is drawn through the tunnel into the abdominal cavity
4. A purse string suture with 2 or 3 metric polydioxanone is preplaced in the fundic portion of the gastric wall and a stab incision made within the suture into the lumen

5. The Foley catheter is then placed into the stomach, the balloon inflated and the purse string suture tightened
6. Omentum is wrapped around the Foley catheter and the purse string suture passed through the abdominal wall for added security
7. The Foley catheter is placed under traction to draw the stomach into firm contact with the abdominal wall and is fixed in place externally either with a Chinese friction finger trap suture pattern or by means of zinc oxide butterfly tapes.

The burn patient's nutritional requirements can be estimated and the diet should provide at least 4 g of protein per 100 kcal in dogs and 6 g per 100 kcal in cats. The injured patient should be fed at least 1.5 times its resting energy requirement (RER). The RER can be calculated using appropriate formulae:

- Patient of 2–45 kg body weight:
  RER (kcal) = 30 x BW + 70
- Patient <2 kg or >45 kg body weight:
  RER (kcal) = 70 x $BW^{0.75}$

Management of the burn wound
The extent of the injuries can be assessed rapidly by the 'Rule of Nine' (see Figure 12.16) and wound management instituted. The goals of wound management are:

- To prevent further thermal injury
- To minimize contamination and infection
- To remove dead tissue
- Reconstruction.

Surgical debridement
Though topical dressings are beneficial in burn wound management, it is current practice to debride large or deep wounds at an early stage. This helps to minimize infection rates by minimizing eschar formation. The aim is to graft or reconstruct the wound as soon as possible. If closure following debridement is not possible, then the site should be treated as an open wound. Such an approach is associated with high success rates in human patients.

Two basic techniques for burn wound debridement (escharotomy) are described in humans: tangential and fascial. Tangential debridement is associated with increased blood loss and involves 'shaving' the dead tissue away from the surface. With most deep wounds it is preferable to perform fascial debridement which is, essentially, an *en bloc* resection of the dead tissues down to healthy tissue (see Chapter 5).

Dressings
Once debrided, burn wounds are best managed by the use of dressings. Dressings should maintain a moist wound environment and be non-adherent (see Chapter 5). In humans there is a move towards using biological dressings such as freeze-dried porcine xenografts or cultured keratinocytes.

There is considerable debate as to the efficacy of topical antimicrobials in burn patients. Some authors advise their immediate use whilst others wait until there is clinical evidence of infection. The most commonly used agent to this effect is silver sulphadiazine 1% cream, which has a broad spectrum of activity against Gram-positive and Gram-negative bacteria as well as *Candida* spp. Systemic antibiotics should not be used until an infection is found to be present and should be chosen based on the results of microbial culture and sensitivity tests.

PROJECTILE INJURIES

In the UK high powered gunshot injuries are relatively uncommon in dogs and cats. It is, however, common to find airgun pellets as incidental findings in cats and shotgun pellets in working gundogs (Figure 12.17). Ballistic injuries vary, depending on the shape, mass, stability, and velocity of the bullet/pellet and the degree of fragmentation created within a wound. All penetrating injuries of this type will be contaminated and must be debrided aggressively.

There are two types of bullet wound: those caused by high-velocity bullets and those caused by low-velocity bullets. The degree and extent of damage caused varies considerably between them (see also Chapter 2).

High-velocity bullets have a huge amount of energy, and are fired with velocities of 800–1000 m/s. When such bullets enter tissue they cause extensive damage through cavitation and shock waves. Such cavities may be 30–40 times greater than the diameter of the bullet (Figure 12.18). Once the bullet has passed through the animal, the cavity will collapse; due to the subatmospheric pressure present it will suck air, debris, hair and bacteria into the wound. Such injuries have the capacity to produce large

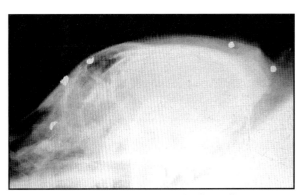

Figure 12.17: *Radiograph showing shotgun pellets as an incidental finding in a working gundog.*

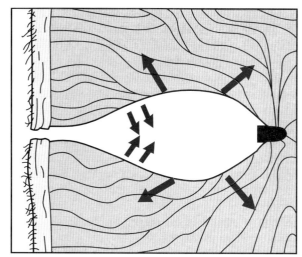

Figure 12.18: Tissue cavity produced by a high-velocity bullet. The arrows indicate the direction and magnitude of expended kinetic energy.

amounts of dead and devitalized, contaminated tissue. The amount of damage depends on the tissue involved. Homogenous structures such as liver or muscle are very sensitive to damage, whereas lung is relatively resistant. Bone, because of its inelastic nature, tends to shatter.

Low-velocity bullets are relatively heavy and designed for use in hand guns. They travel at 200–300 m/s, have relatively low kinetic energy and are usually used at a range of less than 100 m. These bullets tend to bore a hole through tissue and only damage those tissues with which they are in direct contact. They cause life-threatening problems only when vital tissues such as blood vessels are in their path. Their path through the body can be very unpredictable, with no relationship between entry and exit holes, as they may be deflected by organs such as the liver or spleen (Figure 12.19).

Shotgun injuries in working gundogs can be an incidental finding when the patient is radiographed for another complaint. Usually such penetration occurs outside the effective range of most shotguns (30–40 m), with the pellets only entering the subcutaneous and deep fascial layers where they cause little or no harm. Occasionally dogs may be shot at closer range, allowing the pellets to penetrate deep into the body; if they are shot from extremely close range there will be extensive tissue damage over a relatively wide area.

Wound management

All ballistic wounds are grossly contaminated, with potential for large amounts of devitalized tissue, therefore all such wounds should be explored and debrided wherever possible. The entry and exit wounds should be located, explored and debrided. Bullets that are relatively superficial should be removed, although those which are inaccessible are probably best left

unless they involve a vital structure. The majority of low- and high-velocity bullet wounds will, in addition to debridement, require open wound management before attempting closure, because of the high level of contamination. This is especially true of high-velocity injuries.

Thoracic ballistic injuries, as in humans, can, following debridement of the superficial wounds, be left unexplored unless there is evidence of haemothorax or tension pneumothorax. Limb injures which involve shattered bone are best addressed by open wound management and application of an external fixator. Gunshot wounds to the neck are frequently associated with lacerations of the trachea or oesophagus which will require prompt repair following debridement. Around 90% of abdominal gunshot wounds will have associated visceral injury and will require extensive surgical exploration.

Confirmation of the need to perform laparotomy can be obtained by abdominocentesis, diagnostic peritoneal lavage and abdominal radiographs. If there is any evidence of haemorrhage, peritonitis, or food or air within the abdominal cavity, surgical exploration should be performed as soon as the patient is stable. If findings are equivocal, radiographs and diagnostic peritoneal lavage should be repeated after 24 hours.

Laparotomy

Exploratory laparotomy should be thorough and well planned, with the patient clipped and prepared for extension of the incision into the thorax if necessary. Any major haemorrhage should be dealt with first, then a systematic exploration is carried out for evidence of lacerations. The examination should start with the diaphragm and liver, followed by examination of the gastrointestinal tract in its whole length running from the stomach caudal to the descending colon. It is also important to assess the pancreas, spleen, kidneys, ureter and bladder. Small single lacerations of the viscera should be debrided and closed. Large defects may

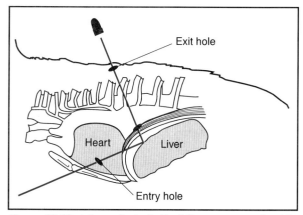

Figure 12.19: A low-velocity bullet follows an unpredictable path. The entry point is on the lateral thorax; following ricochet from the liver, this bullet exits dorsally.

require partial excision of tissue, such as partial hepatic lobectomy, splenectomy, nephrectomy or enterectomy. If there are multiple lacerations of the intestinal tract it may not be possible to resect all affected areas and multiple serosal patching should be performed. If there has been extensive contamination of the peritoneal cavity, open abdominal drainage should be considered.

VASCULAR AUGMENTATION OF WOUND BEDS USING THE OMENTUM

The double peritoneal sheet of the bursal omentum has been used to advantage clinically since 1896 and has gained widespread use in human and veterinary surgery. It has classically been used to seal and repair intra-abdominal structures, and in recent years has been used extra-abdominally as a pedicle graft.

Omentum is a mesothelial membrane and its surgical manipulation relies on its extremely rich vascular and lymphatic supply. The omentum can function in the presence of infection, induce vascularization and adhere to tissues. Omentum mobilizes large numbers of macrophages, mast cells and lymphocytes, which release cytokines that modulate and induce the healing process. These white cells are able to exit the omental lymphatics via 'milk spots' or omental lymphoid organs (OLO) which are aggregates of blind bulbous lymphatic capillaries.

In veterinary surgery, omentum can be used: to aid reconstruction of wounded tissue; to provide drainage of lymphoedema; to seal abdominal (and thoracic) viscera (Hosgood, 1990); and to aid in the management of prostatic abscesses (White and Williams, 1995) and retention cysts (Bray *et al.*, 1997). The omentum can be used surgically as a double or single leaf, both within and outside the abdominal cavity.

Creating an omental pedicle

An omental pedicle is created by detaching the dorsal omental leaf from the pancreas and the spleen (Figure 12.20), thus doubling the length of available omentum. Lengthening the omentum in this way allows it to be used from the axilla to the proximal hindlimbs (Ross and Pardo, 1993).

Occasionally it may be useful to create a pedicle which reaches the distal forelimbs, hindlimbs or the head of an animal. In such cases the omentum is incised in an inverted 'L' shape, starting immediately caudal to the gastrosplenic ligament (Figure 12.21). In most cases it is sufficient to extend only the dorsal portion.

Use of omental pedicles

Omentum can be used in managing chronic non-healing wounds in two ways. One relies on primary wound closure over the site (Brockman *et al.*, 1996) and the other uses omentum as a vascular bed for a free skin graft (Smith *et al.*, 1995).

Omentum is readily used to manage chronic non-healing inguinal and axillary wounds in cats (Brockman *et al.*, 1996; Lascelles *et al.*, 1998) (Figure 12.22). In cats it is essential to rule out any underlying cause (e.g. feline leukaemia virus or feline immunodeficiency virus infection) prior to undertaking surgery.

1. The non-healing wound is preferably excised and a laparotomy (either midline or paracostal) performed
2. Omentum is exteriorized (Figure 12.22b) and a pedicle created of suitable length to reach the wound

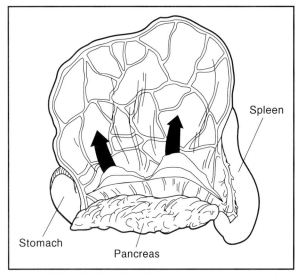

Figure 12.20: *The dorsal leaf of the omentum is detached from the pancreas and spleen. Omental and splenic vessels are ligated as necessary.*

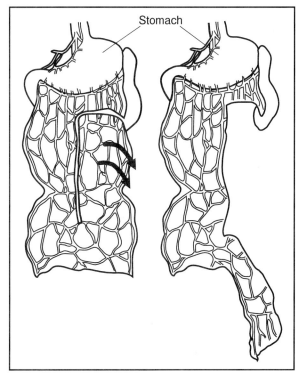

Figure 12.21: *Inverted 'L' extension of the omentum.*

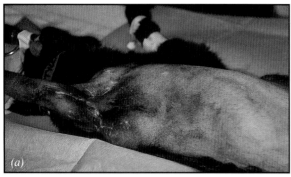

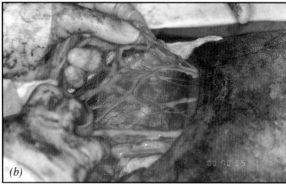

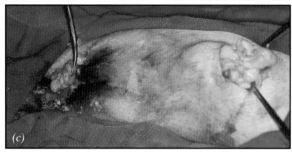

Figure 12.22: (a) A chronic non-healing axillary wound in a cat. (b) Omentum is exteriorized via a paracostal incision. (c) The omentum is drawn very gently through a subcutaneous tunnel, to the axillary wound.

3. A subcutaneous tunnel is created from the laparotomy wound to the non-healing wound site. The omentum is then drawn very gently through the tunnel (Figure 12.22c). Great care must be taken in handling omentum, and its vascular pedicle must not be rotated as this may compromise its blood supply and lymphatics
4. The laparotomy wound is closed and the exit hole for the omentum should be large enough so as to cause no vascular damage while ensuring that visceral herniation does not occur
5. The omentum is sutured into the chronic wound site with simple interrupted absorbable 2 metric sutures, avoiding the blood and lymph vessels
6. Skin is then mobilized over the wound and closed in a routine fashion.

Omentum or muscle (see Chapter 10) can be used to aid reconstruction where large tissue deficits have been created following trauma or radical oncological resections. An example of this is chest wall reconstruction following removal of three or more ribs in the management of a rib-based tumour. The large thoracic defect is initially stabilized by means of synthetic non-absorbable mesh. This is either reinforced by mobilization of the latissimus dorsi muscle or by an omental pedicle. Both types of reinforcement serve to help seal the thoracic wall and to provide a bed over which the skin deficit can be closed.

Full thickness wounds that cannot be closed conventionally can be managed by placement of omentum into the wound bed (Smith *et al.*, 1995). Following aggressive debridement and early wound management an omental pedicle is exteriorized via a paracostal incision, passed through a subcutaneous tunnel, and sutured with simple interrupted absorbable sutures to the bed of the wound. The omentum is then dressed as for an open wound for up to 14 days when it is deemed suitable as a granulated bed for application of a free meshed skin graft (see Chapter 9).

For chronic non-healing wounds or for large defects which appear to have non-viable wound beds (which would not support free skin grafting), creating and exteriorizing an omental pedicle should be considered. This is a readily performed technique and survival of the omentum is excellent as long as it is handled gently.

REFERENCES

Bray JP, White RAS and Williams JM (1997) Partial resection and omentalization: a new technique for management of prostatic retention cysts in dogs. *Veterinary Surgery* **26**, 202–209

Brockman DJ, Pardo AD, Conzemius MG, Cabell LM and Trout NJ (1996) Omentum enhanced reconstruction of chronic non-healing wounds in cats: techniques and clinical use. *Veterinary Surgery* **25**, 99–104

Harkin KR, Walshaw R and Mullaney TP (1996) Association of perianal fistula and colitis in the German shepherd dog: response to high dose prednisone and dietary therapy. *Journal of the American Animal Hospital Association* **32**, 515–520

Hosgood G (1990) The omentum – the forgotten organ – physiology and potential surgical applications in dogs and cats. *Compendium on Continuing Education for the Practicing Veterinarian* **12**, 45–51

Lascelles BDX, Davison L, Dunning M, Bray JP and White RAS (1998) Use of omental pedicle grafts in the management of non-healing axillary wounds in 10 cats. *Journal of Small Animal Practice* **39**, 475–480

Mathews KA, Ayres SA, Tano CA, Riley SM, Sukhiani HR and Adams C (1997) Cyclosporin treatment of perianal fistulas in dogs. *Canadian Veterinary Journal* **38**, 39–41

Pavletic M (1993) *Atlas of Small Animal Reconstructive Surgery.* Lippincott, Philadelphia

Ross WE and Pardo AD (1993) Evaluation of an omental pedicle extension technique in the dog. *Veterinary Surgery* **22**, 37–43

Smith BA, Hosgood G and Hedlund CS (1995) Omental pedicle used to manage a large dorsal wound in a dog. *Journal of Small Animal Practice* **36**, 267–270

Swaim SF and Henderson RA (1997) *Small Animal Wound Management, 2nd edn.* Williams and Wilkins, Baltimore

Westaby S (1989) *Trauma: Pathogenesis and Treatment.* Heinemann, Oxford

White RAS and Lane JG (1988) Pharyngeal stick penetration injuries in the dog. *Journal of Small Animal Practice* **29**, 13–35

White RAS and Williams JM (1995) Intracapsular prostatic omentalization – a new technique for management of prostatic abscesses in dogs. *Veterinary Surgery* **24**, 390–395

CHAPTER THIRTEEN

Complications of Wound Healing

Audrey Remedios

INTRODUCTION

Wound healing is an extremely complicated process that proceeds along four basic and sequential steps:

- Inflammation
- Epithelialization
- Contraction
- Collagen formation.

These phases are interrelated and influenced by factors such as the local wound environment and patient health, which can delay and prevent normal healing. In addition, the application or misapplication of basic surgical principles will also influence healing. Technical considerations, including the use of sharp incisions, atraumatic tissue handling, minimal dissection, adequate debridement, achieving haemostasis and appropriate wound closure, all promote successful wound repair. If these are not adhered to, complications occur. Although most wound complications are not life-threatening, they involve prolonged periods of animal discomfort and veterinary care, and increased costs to owners.

POSTOPERATIVE HAEMORRHAGE AND HAEMATOMAS

Surgical incisions involve the disruption of blood vessels with an initial tissue response of vasoconstriction. However, in the immediate postoperative period, vasodilation, bleeding and haematoma formation can occur. Overt incisional haemorrhage is a burden in patient management, but is usually a minor complication. Haematoma formation, however, can predispose to wound infection, cause discomfort, and prevent healing of reconstructive tissues (e.g. skin grafts) on to wound beds.

Prevention of haemorrhage and subsequent haematoma formation is more prudent than postoperative treatment. During surgery, using appropriately sized ligatures or electrocautery can decrease haemorrhage. Minimizing the amount of subcutaneous dissection will also prevent the accumulation of blood within a defined space. Postoperatively, minor incisional oozing can be controlled with direct manual pressure for 10–15 minutes. However, moderate to severe bleeding will require the application of pressure bandages or surgical ligation of the offending vessels. Once haematoma formation is evident, resolution may be accelerated by the application of warm compresses on to the affected area for 10 minutes, three times a day. Dissipation of the haematoma generally requires approximately 7 days.

SEROMAS

Creation of dead space, either through trauma or by surgical dissection, can result in the accumulation of sterile fluid within the subcutaneous space, a seroma. This fluid tends to form in areas that have redundant, loosely attached skin (Figure 13.1) and are associated with excessive motion (shoulder, axilla and dorsum). Other than the presence of fluid, seromas are associated with few clinical signs. They are not painful, erythematous, oedematous or associated with incisional dehiscence. In fact, seromas most often are a source of owner anxiety, rather than patient discomfort. In some specialized reconstructive procedures, such as skin grafting, seroma formation can be detrimental to the critical adherence of the tissue to the wound bed. Seromas will also delay the ultimate healing of affected tissues.

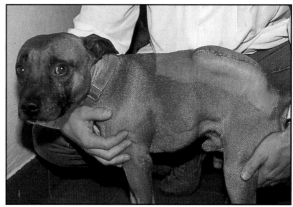

Figure 13.1: Redundant and loosely attached skin predispose the dorsum to seroma formation after surgery. Areas that are associated with excessive motion, and procedures that create extensive dead space, also contribute to fluid accumulation within the subcutaneous space.

Differentiation from abscesses

Seromas must be differentiated from subcutaneous abscesses. Seroma formation can be distinguished from an incisional abscess clinically. Whereas seromas are associated with minimal clinical signs, abscesses provoke intense local inflammation. Thus, abscesses are associated with local skin erythema, oedema, heat, incisional dehiscence, fever and pain. Veterinary surgeons should rely on their clinical skills and judgement to distinguish between seromas and abscesses. Inexperience and a dubious nature may propel individuals to aspirate the seroma contents and examine the fluid. In this situation, it is very easy to convert a pre-existing seroma into an abscess. Should such an impulse be followed, strict aseptic protocol must be applied to minimize complications. The area should be shaved and surgically prepared. The operator should wear sterile gloves and use a sterile syringe and needle to avoid inoculating bacteria into the seroma. Aspirated seromas should be monitored daily to diagnose any untoward complications.

Prevention

Prevention of seroma formation is accomplished by practising gentle tissue handling and eliminating dead space. Surgeries that involve extensive soft tissue dissection and mobilization, such as regional mastectomies and skin flap transfers, will create large amounts of dead space. Subcutaneous sutures, active or passive drains, and bandages are techniques that can be used individually, or in combination, to decrease seroma formation. Although all of these could be applied in clean surgical procedures, the use of buried suture material in clean–contaminated cases should be avoided. In these situations, drains and bandages are preferable. Open system drains (e.g. Penrose drains) should always be covered with bandages to avoid ascending infection.

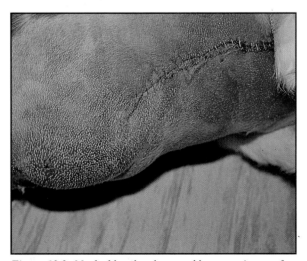

Figure 13.2: *Marked local oedema and hyperaemia are often associated with surgeries that involve extensive subcutaneous dissection, such as regional mastectomies.*

Treatment

Seromas that occur after surgery usually do not require intervention. Attempts at aspiration are futile and risk contaminating a sterile environment. Similarly, drain placement often results in recurrence after drain removal and predisposes to iatrogenic infection. Seromas do resolve spontaneously, but this process may require 2–3 weeks.

OEDEMA

Early wound healing is associated with the process of inflammation. During this process, vascular and lymphatic obstruction and the presence of cell- and plasma-derived mediators result in the exudation of fluid into the interstitial subcutaneous space (oedema formation). Traumatic wounds generally manifest more oedema than surgical wounds. However, depending on the extent of dissection and the nature of the procedure, surgical wounds can also appear oedematous in the first 3–4 days after surgery. Regional mastectomies, for example, often result in marked peri-incisional oedema formation (Figure 13.2).

Some reconstructive procedures, such as skin flaps and grafts, are also associated with marked postoperative oedema. The reverse saphenous skin flap, which depends on a reversal of blood flow through the cranial and caudal branches of the saphenous artery and medial saphenous vein, is particularly susceptible to oedema and congestion. Oedema formation in these flaps will be prolonged for up to 2 weeks after flap transfer. Skin grafts are associated with oedema during the stage of plasmatic imbibition, reaching a maximum at 2–3 days after harvest.

Large skin wounds of the distal limbs which are managed with second intention healing can also result in impaired lymphatic and venous drainage, and oedema formation. Especially when wounds exceed 50% of the circumferential limb diameter, the tension created by wound contracture creates a tourniquet effect and distal limb swelling.

Postoperative oedema can be treated using compression bandages. As loosening occurs, new bandages need to be applied daily to maintain even pressure. The application of warm compresses to the affected area 3-4 times daily promotes circulation and decreases oedema formation. If oedema is confined to the limbs, active movement increases circulation and promotes lymphatic and venous return.

WOUND DEHISCENCE

Dehiscence is defined as the breakdown of a surgically closed wound. Immediately after closure, a problem incision may be erythematous, oedematous or painful. Often, a serosanguineous discharge is associated with

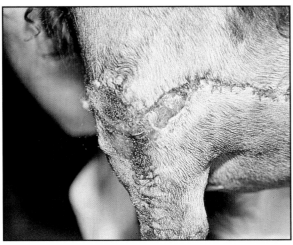

Figure 13.3: Incisional dehiscence is glaringly evident 3–5 days after surgery.

the wound edges. Generally, irrefutable evidence of incisional breakdown becomes apparent at 3–5 days after surgery. Areas of non-viable necrotic tissue may also be evident at that time (Figure 13.3).

Wound dehiscence is rarely due to an intrinsic inability to heal; rather, problems associated with surgical judgement or technique and the wound bed are incriminated. Probably the most common reason for dehiscence after closure of a traumatic wound is incomplete debridement of contaminated material and necrotic tissue. As all traumatic wounds are contaminated, a thorough assessment of the cause and nature of the wound must be performed initially.

Crush injuries

Wounds that are associated with crush injuries, such as dog bites and vehicular degloving, and wounds that are grossly contaminated with debris, should not be closed primarily. These injuries require at least 2–3 days of daily open wound management (debridement and lavage; see Chapter 5) in order to assess local blood supply and to be sure that non-viable or contaminated tissues have been removed. If surgical closure is attempted in these cases, then the underlying necrosis and infection will undoubtedly lead to wound dehiscence.

Sharp lacerations

Wounds that are a result of sharp lacerations still require stringent initial assessment prior to primary closure. Here, the surgeon must adhere to sterile principles regarding patient preparation and instrument preparation. The wound should be evaluated and prepared in a surgical fashion, all suspect tissue must be debrided to healthy, bleeding edges, and liberal lavage should be performed. It is best to avoid burying deep and subcutaneous sutures in these clean/contaminated wounds, as they can serve as a nidus of infection. Using drains or pressure bandages to eliminate dead space is more appropriate upon primary or delayed primary closure of traumatic wounds.

Incisions

Incisions, of either traumatic or surgical origin, can also break down due to inappropriate surgical techniques. In deep layers, incisional dehiscence will lead to herniation of internal contents. Breakdown after closure of the abdominal wall is probably the most common and most serious scenario. Several factors can result in abdominal herniation:

- The size and choice of suture material must be appropriate. Abdominal incisions are closed with 3-0 suture material in cats and small breed dogs, 2-0 in medium-sized dogs, 0 in large breed dogs, and 1 in giant dogs. Recommended suture materials include polyglycolic acid, polyglactin 910, and polydioxanone.
- It is especially important to ensure that square knots are created rather than 'granny' or slip knots. Generally, the minimum number of throws necessary to make secure simple interrupted knots is three for polyglycolic acid or polyglactin 910, and four for polydioxanone. Secure square knots to start and finish a simple continuous pattern should have at least six throws.
- Probably the most common cause of abdominal wall dehiscence is the misjudgement and lack of recognition of the layer of strength at the time of closure. Whether an abdominal incision is midline or paramedian, the layer of strength is the external leaf of the rectus sheath. Studies have shown that the strength of incisions closed by suturing the internal and external rectus sheaths is similar to that of the external sheath alone (Rosin and Richardson, 1987). In addition, closure of the peritoneum is unnecessary and predisposes to adhesion formation. Typically, abdominal wall dehiscence arises from inadvertent closure of the subcutaneous layer instead of the external rectus sheath. Especially in large breed or obese dogs, the delineation between the external sheath and subcutaneous tissue is subtle. The surgeon must strive to separate these layers to ensure appropriate closure.

Superficial wounds

Closure of superficial wound layers also requires the application of appropriate surgical techniques in order to minimize the risk of dehiscence. Excessive tension on the suture line is a common cause of cutaneous dehiscence. In dogs and cats, the abundance of loose skin in the thoracic and abdominal regions allows for the closure of most wounds by undermining and advancing the wound's edges with walking subcutaneous sutures (see Chapter 7). In some cases, use of tension relieving suture patterns, such as far-near-near-far or far-far-near-near, may be necessary to appose the skin edges.

Wounds associated with the limbs can pose problems for closure, however. Where the wound is less than one third of the limb circumference, multiple punctate releasing incisions can be made in a parallel fashion in the adjacent skin (Figure 13.4). When the primary incision is closed, these punctate incisions will expand to form a mesh and minimize tension. The small multiple punctate incisions are left to heal by second intention. Large wounds involving the limbs often require skin flaps or grafts to provide additional soft tissue coverage (see Chapter 9).

Management

When wound dehiscence does occur, management must first be directed at identifying any contributing factors. In traumatic wounds, residual contamination or necrotic tissue is often the cause of incisional problems. Such incisions should be opened and assessed thoroughly. Wound debridement and lavage should be performed. If doubt remains as to tissue viability or degree of contamination, then open wound management should be continued for 2–3 days prior to closure. Incisional herniations require surgery to explore the hernia contents and apply appropriate surgical techniques to affect successful closure. Since closure of the subcutaneous layer instead of the external rectus

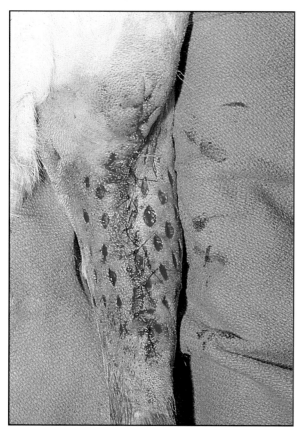

Figure 13.4: *One method of overcoming excessive skin tension on the suture line is the use of multiple punctate releasing incisions. The 0.5 cm parallel skin incisions are made in staggered rows approximately 2 cm apart. When undermined, these incisions will expand to form a mesh and facilitate skin closure.*

sheath is a common surgical error, an effort must be made to identify the layer of strength and to close it with appropriate suture material. Incisions that break down because of excessive skin tension can be treated as open wounds, allowing for second intention healing to occur, or application of other surgical techniques, such as skin flaps and grafts may be necessary.

INFECTION

A break in the skin barrier, from either trauma or surgery, inevitably leads to bacterial contamination. Postoperative infection has been documented to occur in approximately 5% of all small animal surgical procedures and in 2.5% of clean surgeries (Vasseur, 1988). In most patients, host defence systems will phagocytose microbes and prevent infection. However, when bacterial numbers exceed a critical level ($>10^6$ organisms per gram of tissue), infection will occur. Several factors, including local wound conditions, the type of bacteria involved and the status of the patient, may dampen normal defence mechanisms and predispose to infection. In traumatic wounds, the most common source of infection is the presence of non-viable tissue.

Normally, after an incision or laceration, neutrophils migrate to the wound and engulf and destroy microbes. Macrophage recruitment occurs later and enhances neutrophil phagocytosis. Any local condition that prevents the ability of these cells to contact and kill bacteria will potentiate infection. Haematoma or seroma formation will prevent the adherence of neutrophils to the bacterial cell walls and may also serve as a substrate for microbial growth. Implantation of foreign bodies, such as drains and sutures, will decrease the number of bacteria necessary to cause an infection. Animals that are immunocompromised because of pre-existing diseases (hyperadrenocorticism, diabetes mellitus, or neoplasia), or because of exogenous medications (corticosteroids) are more susceptible to infections. Undeveloped or senescent resistance processes may also affect the very young or old animal.

Bacterial species

The kind of bacteria affecting a wound will influence greatly the risk of infection. In dogs, soft tissue infections not involving the gastrointestinal system are usually associated with *Staphylococcus* spp. However, *Escherichia coli* and anaerobic bacteria, such as *Bacteroides* and *Clostridium*, frequently contaminate wounds that are located near the portals of the alimentary tract. In cats, *Pasteurella* is the most common isolate from soft tissue infections. Some bacteria which elaborate endotoxins, such as *E. coli*, cause direct cellular toxicity and prevent phagocytosis by host defence cells. Others, including *Clostridium*, may produce exotoxins that cause a more rapid onset of infection with fewer bacterial numbers.

Clinical signs

The clinical signs of a wound infection usually manifest at 2–3 days after surgery. The animal may show systemic signs of illness, such as inactivity and inappetence, or have an elevated body temperature. More often, skin wounds are associated with local changes only. The affected area is warm, erythematous, oedematous and painful. The incision may be gaping and associated with a serosanguinous, mucoid or purulent discharge.

Diagnosis

Should clinical signs suggest a surgical infection then deep aspirates of the wound are recommended to confirm the diagnosis and isolate the offending organisms. To avoid inadvertent contamination, a sterile surgical preparation of the skin should be performed prior to aspiration. The operator should also wear sterile gloves and use sterile implements. The specimen is then examined cytologically and cultured for aerobic and anaerobic bacteria.

Prevention

Prevention of infection is more practical and cost-efficient than treating postoperative complications. In clean surgeries, minimizing bacterial contamination from the patient and adhering to sound surgical technique are important factors in preventing wound infection. Avoidance of bacterial contamination is implemented by controlling the operating room environment, appropriate patient preparation, and constant vigilance by the surgeon.

The operating room

Many modern surgical theatres are equipped with unidirectional or laminar flow ventilation systems that limit airborne contamination. Although the costs associated with such engineering designs are prohibitive for most private practices, there are some rules that can be implemented to help decrease infection:

- The surgical theatre should be an enclosed area that is isolated from noise and 'traffic'
- A separate area should serve for anaesthesia induction and patient preparation
- 'Traffic' in and out of the operating room should be limited
- Activity and talking should be minimized
- Strict sterilization techniques for instruments must be followed.

Patient preparation

Removal of fur from the surgical area should be extensive and complete, and performed immediately before an operation. Shaving an operative site 24 hours before surgery will increase infection rates by 100% (Alexander *et al.*, 1983). As the skin is an important source of contaminants, appropriate preparation is essential in preventing complications. The skin is prepared with a 5–7 minute scrub using a germicidal detergent, then painted with isopropyl alcohol. In addition, antimicrobial plastic drapes can be used to isolate the surrounding skin from the incised wound.

Scrubbing up

Wearing a clean scrub suit, cap and mask, the veterinary surgeon should perform a 3–5 minute scrub of both hands and forearms. Careful gowning, gloving and draping techniques should be used as these often are sources of transgressions in operating sterility. Punctures in gloves are common (as many as 90%), especially during long surgeries. Although the numbers of microbes are low after a surgical scrub, bacterial contamination will increase during long surgeries and especially once blood contacts the surgeon's hands. The safest practice is to wear two pairs of gloves, with the outer gloves a half size larger. This is especially important in procedures that involve the internal implantation of bone cement, such as total hip replacement.

Surgical technique

The importance of surgical technique and judgement in the prevention of postoperative infection cannot be overemphasized. Even in clean surgeries, the implantation of buried suture predisposes to bacterial growth. Historical studies (Elek and Conen, 1957) have shown that, while more than a million staphylococcal organisms are required to create an infection when inoculated into normal subcutaneous tissue, as few as 100 of the same bacteria can promote infection in the presence of multifilamented suture material (Figure 13.5).

The creation of dead space and the subsequent formation of haematomas or seromas will also enhance infection and dampen local immune responses. In clean surgeries, elimination of dead space is best performed using subcutaneous sutures and bandages. Although there is an attendant risk of infection associated with buried sutures, this must be balanced against the effect of haematoma and seroma formation. In clean–contaminated surgeries and traumatic wounds, use of closed or open drains may be preferable to buried sutures when decreasing dead space.

Prior to closure of any traumatic wound, all devitalized tissue and foreign bodies should be removed. Should any doubt remain as to tissue viability, then the wound should be managed as an open defect, and primary closure delayed for 3–5 days.

Prophylactic antibiotics

The use of prophylactic antibiotics to prevent postoperative infection remains controversial. Clean surgeries, which are associated with low infection rates (2.5%), do not benefit from perioperative administration of antibiotics. Only when the duration of surgery exceeds 90 minutes or when inexperienced operators perform the surgery does prophylaxis reduce infection rate (Vasseur, 1988).

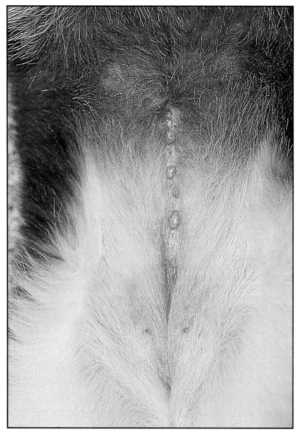

Figure 13.5: Buried sutures are foreign material and can predipose to infection even in clean surgeries, such as a ventral abdominal ovariohysterectomy. Fewer bacteria are required to promote infection following the use of multifilamented suture material.

Clean-contaminated procedures are associated with slightly higher rates of postoperative infection (4.5%) (Vasseur, 1988). In such cases, the degree and source of contamination, and the ability to minimize bacterial numbers during surgery, are important considerations in judging the necessity of prophylactic antibiotics. For example, clinical problems tend to arise only if large amounts of small intestine contents are spilled into the abdomen. However, higher bacterial numbers associated with colonic contents render any spillage more hazardous. Although prophylactic antibiotic administration is indicated in these scenarios, minimizing bacterial numbers through copious lavage is probably the best tactic for decreasing postoperative infection.

If they are used, prophylactic antibiotics are most effective when given preoperatively and continued throughout surgery. Effective therapeutic blood levels are achieved through intravenous administration. If antibiotic administration is delayed for 1-2 hours after contamination has occurred, efficacy is significantly diminished. If given after wound closure, there is no benefit provided by the use of antibiotics. Continuation of antibiotic administration in the postoperative period is of no value and will not decrease infection rates. The choice of antibiotics should be targeted at bacteria that are most likely to be present at the surgical site.

Treatment

Treatment of postoperative infection requires initial consideration as to cause. However, regardless of aetiology, the safest management approach involves surgical exploration of the infected site. The wound must be debrided of all necrotic tissue or foreign bodies. If not performed previously, swabs should be taken for aerobic and anaerobic culture at this time. Copious lavage will aid in reduction of bacterial numbers. Surgical infections are generally not closed primarily but managed as open wounds for several days prior to closure. Antibiotic treatment is based on culture results and is continued for 10-14 days.

DELAYED AND INCOMPLETE WOUND HEALING

Wounds that are left to heal by second intention can be complicated by delayed healing and incomplete epithelialization. Skin defects over loose-skinned areas, such as the thorax and abdomen, are generally not affected. However, wounds that encompass half the circumference of the limbs or greater are at risk for these complications. As the size of a defect increases, tension in the surrounding skin is created which overcomes the contraction of myofibroblasts. Since the myofibroblasts cannot pull the wound edges together,

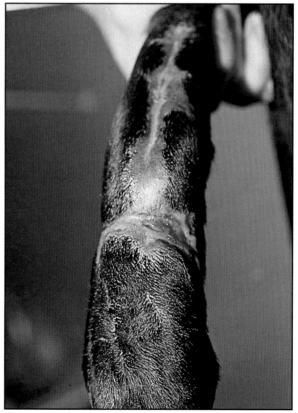

Figure 13.6: Prolonged healing times and wide epithelial scars are often associated with limb wounds managed by second intention healing. This method of treatment is costly and results in thinner, more fragile scar epithelium.

the net effect is to delay and even stop wound contraction. Further healing can occur only by epithelial migration over the wound bed. Epithelial migration begins at the wound edges and moves centripetally. As the defect size increases, the regenerated epithelium becomes thinner and complete coverage may not occur. In addition, scar epithelium is thinner and thus, more prone to injury than normal skin (Figure 13.6). In cases where large wounds involving the limbs are likely to result in prolonged and incomplete healing, reconstructive procedures (skin flaps and grafts) should be performed.

WOUND CONTRACTURE

Wound contracture, especially following second intention healing, can lead to loss or altered function. The contracture of wounds situated over flexor surfaces may lead to decreased range of joint motion and subsequent lameness. Defects involving any orifice (eye, mouth and anus) can result in stenosis and functional deformity. Specialized reconstructive procedures (e.g. Z plasties, advancement flaps; see Chapter 7) can be performed to restore normal function.

REFERENCES

Alexander JW, Fischer JE, Boyajiain M, Palmquist J and Morris MJ (1983) Infuence of hair-removal methods on wound infections. *Archives-of-Surgery* **118**, 347-348

Elek SD and Conen PE (1957) The virulence of Staphylococcus pyogenes for man. A study in the problems of wound infection. *British Journal of Experimental Pathology* **38**, 573-576

Rosin E and Richardson S (1987) Effect of fascial closure technique on strength of healing abdominal incisions in the dog: a biomechanical study. *Veterinary Surgery* **16**, 269-272

Rosin E and Robinson GM (1989) Knot security of suture materials. *Veterinary Surgery* **18**, 269-273

Vasseur PB (1988) Surgical wound infection rates in dogs and cats. *Veterinary Surgery* **17**, 60-64

CHAPTER FOURTEEN

Case Examples

David Fowler and John M. Williams

CASE ONE: 8-year-old spayed female Labrador Retriever cross with a basal cell tumour of the footpad

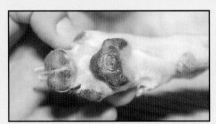
Figure 14.1

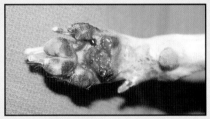
Figure 14.2

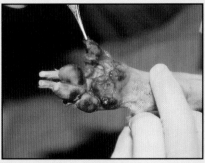
Figure 14.3

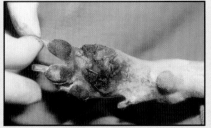
Figure 14.4

History
The bitch was presented with a subtle forelimb lameness attributed to a firm lesion located in the metacarpal footpad of the left forelimb (Figure 14.1).

Assessment and management options
Biopsy of the mass led to a histopathological diagnosis of basal cell tumour. This is a relatively benign tumour in the dog, and resection with minimal margins is usually curative. However, local resection in this case necessitated resection of more than 50% of the metacarpal footpad. Wound breakdown and inadequate resistance to weight-bearing stresses can be anticipated following resection of a large portion of this footpad. Reconstructive options included footpad grafts or digital footpad transposition.

Footpad grafts were considered. However, footpad grafts include only the dermal and epidermal components of the pad. The footpad cushion, which is important in the diffusion of weight-bearing stresses, cannot be transferred with footpad grafts. Therefore, a digital footpad transposition technique was used as the reconstructive option of choice (Figure 14.2).

Treatment
The 3rd and 4th digits bear the majority of the weight-bearing stress of the foot, but loss of the 2nd or 5th digit is associated with little, if any, loss of function. Therefore, the 2nd or 5th digital footpads can be used to provide footpad tissue for transposition to neighbouring locations that are more crucial to weight-bearing function.

In this case, the 5th digital footpad was dissected, using a digital filleting technique (Figure 14.3). The phalangeal bones were excised through a dorsal midline longitudinal incision, taking care to preserve all soft tissues and neurovascular structures. Following removal of the phalangeal bones, a bridging incision was made through the interdigital web, extending from the donor to the recipient site. The digital footpad was then simply transposed on to the recipient wound bed and all incisions closed primarily (Figure 14.4).

In such cases, protection from weight-bearing stresses, using heavily padded bandages and exercise restriction, is required until soft tissue healing is advanced – usually 3 to 4 weeks. Subsequent weight-bearing stresses should be introduced gradually to allow progressive remodelling of the wound.

CASE TWO: Five-year-old female Samoyed with a full thickness burn

History

The bitch was initially presented to the referring veterinary surgeon with a closed pyometra. She was depressed and mildly dehydrated; laboratory assessment revealed profound neutrophilia with a left shift. The bitch was stabilized by administering intravenous balanced electrolyte solution and was started on systemic antibiotics. Subsequent ovariohysterectomy and recovery from anaesthesia were uncomplicated. At the time of suture removal 10 days after surgery, an area of skin necrosis was apparent over the caudal lumbar region. She had been placed on an electric heating pad during ovariohysterectomy and skin necrosis had occurred secondary to thermal injury.

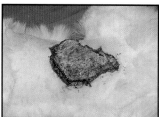

Figure 14.5

Wound assessment

This lesion (Figure 14.5) represented a full thickness burn wound with minimal exudate and no evidence of infection. Debridement of all necrotic tissue with subsequent open wound management was indicated. Reconstruction could be considered once all ongoing tissue necrosis had been controlled.

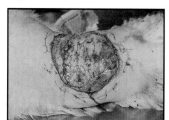

Figure 14.6

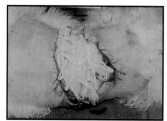

Figure 14.7

Treatment

En bloc debridement of all necrotic skin and subcutaneous tissue was performed (Figure 14.6). The use of sterile instruments and aseptic technique minimized further contamination and decreased the risk of nosocomial infection. Immediate reconstruction was considered. However, as it is often difficult to ascertain the extent of non-viable tissue after initial debridement, a judicious approach was adopted and the wound was managed open, using a wet-to-dry contact layer with a tie-over bolus type dressing (Figure 14.7) A hydrogel rather than an adherent contact dressing could have been considered as an alternative. The bandage was changed daily, and lavage and layered debridement repeated as needed. Antibiotics were not administered.

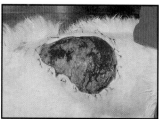

Figure 14.8

Further assessment

Three days after initial debridement, there was no evidence of ongoing tissue necrosis and tissues within the wound were well vascularized (Figure 14.8). The wound was now classified as clean–contaminated, and was appropriate for delayed primary closure.

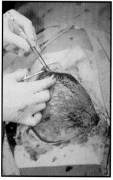

Figure 14.9

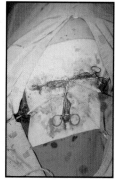

Figure 14.10

Further treatment

A great deal of mobile skin was present on the trunk. Direct suture closure, facilitated by tissue undermining, can be achieved in lesions of this size. Reconstruction was performed under surgically aseptic conditions. Skin surrounding the lesion was undermined deep to the cutaneous trunci muscle to preserve the vascular supply to the skin (Figure 14.9).

Tissues are advanced in the direction of greatest elasticity or distensibility, determined by grasping the skin and attempting advancement in different directions. Backhaus towel clamps were used at key locations to maintain skin edges in apposition during suturing (Figure 14.10).

CASE TWO continues ▶

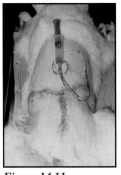

Tissue advancement resulted in the formation of a Y-shaped closure. Tissue apposition was maintained using absorbable suture material placed in a cruciate pattern into subcutaneous tissue along the skin margin.

Walking sutures were not required to achieve tissue apposition, therefore minimizing the amount of buried suture material within the wound. Dead space was managed using a closed suction drain (Figure 14.11), which was removed after 4 days.

Outcome
Subsequent healing was uneventful.

Figure 14.11

CASE THREE: 2-year-old castrated male Domestic Shorthair with a non-healing chronic axillary wound

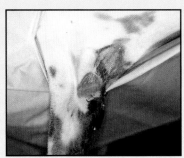

Figure 14.12

History
The cat was presented with a 6-week history of a chronic axillary wound following a leg entrapment in its collar. The wound was 2 cm in diameter, non-healing and with chronic granulation tissue present (Figure 14.12). The cat was negative for both FIV and FeLV.

Management options
Non-healing chronic axillary wounds can be very difficult to manage due to the constant motion at the site. It was therefore decided to use a flap to minimize tension and to utilize omentum to enhance the healing potential of the area. A number of options were available in this case, e.g. advancement flap, a 45 degree transposition flap, or a thoracodorsal axial flap. Omentum provides the necessary angiogenic factors to allow relatively rapid healing.

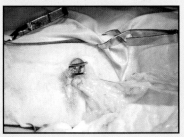

Figure 14.13

Treatment
The cat was clipped and draped for aseptic surgery to allow access to both the axilla and the paracostal area. The wound was excised.

A separate incision was made in the paracostal area to exteriorize the omentum (Figure 14.13); there was no need to carry out omental extension in this case. A subcutaneous tunnel was created between the axilla and the paracostal incision. Omentum was drawn through the tunnel to the axilla (Figure 14.14). A skin incision was made at the proximal end of the axillary wound to release tension. A standard advancement flap was found not to be necessary, due to the elastic nature of the cat's skin. Sutures were only placed in the wound edges; no walking or tacking sutures were used in the body of the flap. The wound was closed in an L shape (Figures 14.15 and 14.16) with simple interrupted sutures of 3 metric monfilament nylon. The

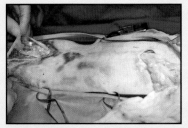

Figure 14.14

paracostal incision through the muscles was partially closed so as not to compromise omental blood supply and the skin incision was closed routinely.

Outcome
Healing in this case was uneventful.

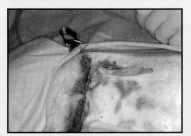

Figure 14.15

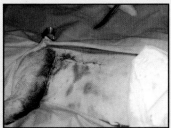

Figure 14.16

CASE FOUR: 3-year-old spayed female Dobermann Pinscher

History
The bitch was presented acutely following a traumatic injury to the forelimb. She had been caught in a grain auger and had suffered a severe laceration/avulsion injury to the flexor surface of the distal radius and ulna.

Initial assessment
The wound was heavily contaminated with soil and grain. The radius was intact, but the ulna had sustained a fracture with segmental bone loss. All major flexor muscles were disrupted with significant loss of tissue. The neurovascular supply to the distal extremity and foot was intact.

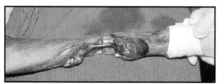

Figure 14.17

Initial treatment
Due to the extent of contamination, immediate reconstruction was considered inappropriate. The bitch was systemically stable, and was placed under general anaesthesia for aggressive local debridement and lavage. The wound was managed open, using a wet-to-dry contact dressing with daily debridement and lavage for 3 days. No further tissue necrosis or foreign contaminants could be identified at that time, and the wound was considered to be clean–contaminated (Figure 14.17).

Further assessment and management options
This was a devastating injury, necessitating complex local reconstruction.

Amputation was considered, but was declined by the owner. Factors considered in selecting an appropriate method of reconstruction included: the presence of exposed bone; extensive loss of soft tissues; and the loss of weight-bearing support provided by the flexor muscles. Carpal arthrodesis was required to provide structural integrity during weight-bearing, but should not be performed in a contaminated wound bed. Therefore, rapid reconstruction of the wound using well vascularized tissue was considered essential for rapid rehabilitation of the wound and to facilitate staged carpal arthrodesis at the earliest opportunity. A free microvascular transfer of the trapezius muscle, resurfaced with a full thickness skin graft was chosen.

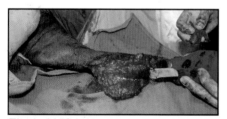

Figure 14.18

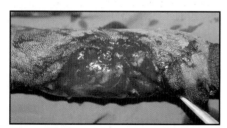

Figure 14.19

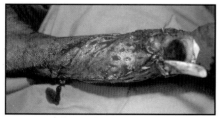

Figure 14.20

Reconstruction
The trapezius muscle is a broad, flat muscle with a dominant vascular pedicle formed by the superficial cervical artery and vein. This muscle is very versatile for use in reconstruction of complex extremity wounds. The muscle was dissected from the lateral cervical region; simultaneously the recipient site was surgically debrided and a suitable recipient artery and vein were identified. The vascular pedicle of the trapezius muscle was then transected and the muscle was moved to the recipient site and inset with several absorbable sutures (Figure 14.18).

Using an operating microscope and standard microvascular technique, the muscle was revascularized by end-to-side anastomosis of the donor artery to the radial artery, and end-to-end anastomosis of the donor vein to the cephalic vein. Successful establishment of blood flow was documented 30 minutes after completion of both anastomoses. Following vascular anastomosis, placement of the flap was completed and dead space deep to the muscle flap was managed using a latex drain (Figure 14.19).

The muscle was immediately resurfaced with a meshed full thickness skin graft (Figure 14.20). The graft was covered with a porous non-adherent contact dressing and was immobilized in a heavily padded splint. Bandage changes were performed daily to allow evaluation of the skin graft and the underlying muscle flap.

CASE FOUR continues ▶

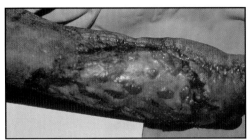

Figure 14.21

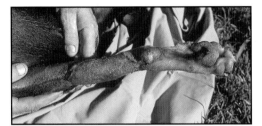

Figure 14.22

Figure 14.21 shows the appearance after 13 days.

Further treatment

Carpal arthrodesis was performed using a dorsal approach to the distal radius, carpus and metacarpus. The articular surfaces of the distal radius and the radiocarpal bone were excised using a saggital bone saw. The intercarpal and carpometacarpal joints were exposed and articular cartilage was removed using a high speed burr.

All joint surfaces were flushed thoroughly and packed with cancellous bone graft harvested from the proximal humerus. The carpus was stabilized in 10 degrees extension, using a 3.5 mm dynamic compression plate.

Outcome

Subsequent healing was uneventful and weight-bearing function was restored, with a satisfactory cosmetic outcome (Figure 14.22).

CASE FIVE: Ten-month-old male German Shepherd cross with a full thickness abrasion

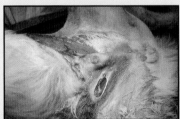

Figure 14.23

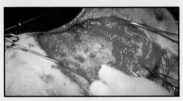

Figure 14.24

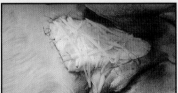

Figure 14.25

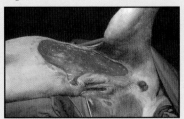

Figure 14.26

History

The dog was presented acutely following a road traffic accident. Intravenous balanced electrolyte solution was initially administered at shock doses. Thorough evaluation revealed no evidence of injury other than an extensive full thickness abrasion type injury involving the skin of the ventral abdominal wall (Figure 14.23). Opioid analgesic agents were administered and the dog was observed for 24 hours prior to initiating specific wound therapy. Although delay of wound debridement can increase the risk of wound infection, general anaesthesia is best delayed until the presence or absence of concomitant injuries is fully assessed.

Initial wound treatment

Layered wound debridement (Figure 14.24) was performed under general anaesthesia. An extensive open wound was present, involving the ventral abdominal wall to the left of the prepuce; a smaller open wound was present to the right of the prepuce. The prepuce itself was spared from injury. The wound was managed using a bolus tie-over dressing with a wet-to-dry contact layer (Figure 14.25). Tie-over dressings are indicated in areas that are otherwise difficult to bandage because of conformation or location. The bandage was changed daily and lavage and debridement were repeated. The contact layer was changed to a hydrogel dressing once ongoing tissue necrosis was controlled. Antibiotics were not used.

Management options

Healthy granulation tissue covered the wound, there was no ongoing tissue necrosis, and wound exudate was minimal by 7 days after injury (Figure 14.26). Management options were considered. Second intention healing was not an option since wound contraction would probably have

CASE FIVE continues ▶

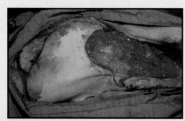

Figure 14.27

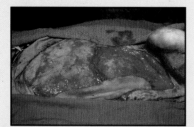

Figure 14.28

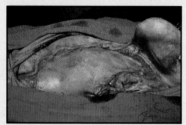

Figure 14.29

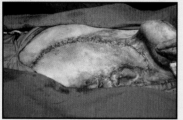

Figure 14.30

resulted in loss of hindlimb mobility due to fibrosis of the inguinal fold, as well as deviation of the prepuce. Local tissue advancement and mesh expansion are difficult in this location, since skin is only available from the cranial wound margin. Skin grafts can be used in this location, but control of motion and shear stresses acting on the graft during healing are difficult to control. As the goal was to redistribute tension away from critical structures (the prepuce and inguinal fold) and into areas where tension is better tolerated, a rotation subdermal plexus flap, based on the lateral thorax, was chosen for reconstruction in this dog (Figure 14.27).

Treatment

Ideally, the arc of incision of a rotation flap should be approximately four times the distance the flap is moved, but the size of the defect in this dog precluded a flap of this dimension. Careful preoperative planning was required to ensure that flap viability would be maintained and that the flap could be rotated into the desired position. The base of the rotation flap in this case incorporated the cranial superficial epigastric artery and vein, ensuring a relatively robust vascular supply. Retraction of the defect and contraction of the flap occurred following dissection of the rotation flap (Figure 14.28).

The advancing tip of the rotation flap was first sutured to the most distant aspect of the defect, using a subcutaneous absorbable suture. The length of the flap was then sutured to the length of the donor and recipient site defects by first placing a single suture at the midpoints of both cutaneous margins. Additional sutures were placed at the midpoints of the two smaller resulting defects. By placing sutures in this fashion, tension was equally distributed throughout the incisional margin (Figure 14.29). Walking sutures are avoided in subdermal plexus flaps, since they can damage the blood supply.

Outcome

The completed closure revealed reconstruction of the entire wound with minimal effect on the prepuce or inguinal fold (Figure 14.30).

CASE SIX: 4-year-old castrated male crossbreed dog with a degloving wound of the proximal antebrachium

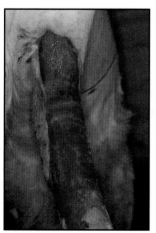

Figure 14.31

History

The dog was involved in a road traffic accident and subsequently developed severe swelling of the left foreleg from the elbow distally. Radiographs made at the time revealed no evidence of bone damage. The swelling persisted for 10 days, when a serosanguinous discharge was noted from the elbow area. The skin on the cranial aspect of the limb sloughed at this time. The area was debrided and managed as an open wound.

At presentation at the referral clinic (3 weeks post injury) a severe skin deficit was noted from the distal humerus to the proximal third of the antebrachium. The wound was granulating and re-epithelializing, with a deep pocket undermining the proximomedial aspect (Figure 14.31). Contracture was noted and there was little, if any, joint movement. Radiographs taken at this time revealed no bone or joint changes. The wound surface and pocket were swabbed; culture revealed no evidence of bacteria.

CASE SIX continues ▶

Assessment and management options

The main concern in managing this wound was to maintain/restore limb function. It was therefore necessary to excise the granulating tissue and to reconstruct. Due to the potential mobility of the wound a free skin graft was not felt to be appropriate and a pedicled skin flap was considered. Due to the large distal extent of this wound, skin viability of the flap was thought to be best served using an axial pattern flap. In this area either an omocervical or thoracodorsal flap could be considered. Either flap would need to be of the extended type, which pass across the patient's midline to the opposite scapula. It is important to note that such an 'extended'

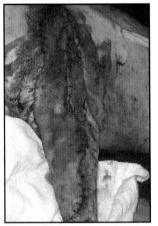

Figure 14.32

excision goes well beyond the boundaries of the flap's primary angiosome; the 'extended' portion of this flap should in fact be considered a subdermal plexus flap in terms of its perfusion and reliability. Due to the large epithelialized pocket on the craniomedial aspect of the wound, which might have interfered with the omocervical blood supply, a thoracodorsal flap was chosen.

Treatment

The chronic granulating tissue and epithelial pockets were excised and a thoracodorsal artery-based flap was raised, with the distal extremity of the flap at the contralateral acromion. This allowed complete coverage of the excised wound (Figure 14.32). Donor site closure was routine, due to the elastic nature of the skin over the dorsum. Penrose drains were placed to manage dead space. The flap achieved excellent coverage of the wound. Due to the nature of the dog it was necessary to dress the wound.

Postoperative assessment and further management

Five days post surgery it was clear that the distal extremity of the flap was not vascularized. By day 7 it was grossly necrotic (Figure 14.33). The patient was taken back to the theatre and the ischaemic area debrided.

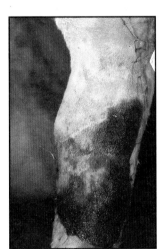

Figure 14.33

As there was concern that infection was present deep to the ischaemic portion of the flap, the distal portion of the flap was managed as an open wound (wet-to-dry dressings) for 5 days to allow granulation tissue to develop, then a free skin graft was applied. The graft donor site was the flank of the dog, which healed without complications. The graft was applied as a meshed full thickness graft and dressed with a non-adherent dressing. Graft immobilization proved very difficult in this case due to the patient's temperament and repeated traumatization of the dressings. Eventually an area on the distal antebrachium was allowed to heal by secondary intention due to free skin graft failure (Figure 14.34). Note the fragile appearance of the covering epithelium. It was decided not to pursue further reconstruction at this time as the dog was using the limb well.

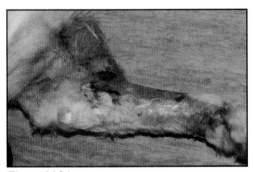

Figure 14.34

Re-presentation

The dog was re-presented 2 years later due to extensive self-trauma to the fragile re-epithelialized area.

Assessment and management options

The priority at this time was wound coverage to protect the delicate epithelium. It was decided that the best option was to repeat a free skin graft following resection of the epithelial tissues. The resected tissue was submitted for histological evaluation to ensure that no neoplastic tissue was present.

Treatment

Following excision, the recipient site was managed as an open wound with a hydrogel and an absorptive foam dressing. After 5 days a free skin graft was applied (as before). The wound was dressed for 5 days

CASE SIX continues ▶

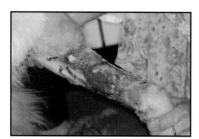

Figure 14.35

initially, after which time the graft was found to be infected (Figure 14.35). Culture of a swab sample showed haemolytic staphylococci; antibiosis was instituted based on the results of *in vitro* sensitivity testing.

After 14 days of antibiotic therapy a third skin graft was applied.

Outcome

The third skin graft 'took', though the grafted area was denuded of hair in comparison to the surrounding skin (Figure 14.36).

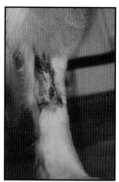

Figure 14.36

CASE SEVEN: 8-year-old male Collie cross with a perineal hernia

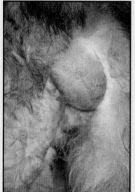

Figure 14.37

History

The dog was presented to the hospital with a complaint of tenesmus of several months. Severity of clinical signs had worsened progressively and the owner had noticed an enlarging 'bulge' located to the right side of the anus (Figure 14.37). The dog had an incidental history of having suffered pelvic fracture at 5 years of age.

Assessment and management options

Rectal examination revealed a loss of support from the perineal diaphragm on the right side, consistent with a diagnosis of perineal hernia. The prostate gland was non-painful but was moderately and symmetrically enlarged. Perineal hernias typically occur in intact male dogs and their development is thought to be hormonally dependent. Castration is routinely recommended as part of the surgical management of this problem. In addition, reconstruction of the perineal diaphragm is essential to provide support to the rectal wall during elimination. The preferred option for reconstruction of the perineal diaphragm is through the use of a pedicled internal obturator muscle flap. In this case, the integrity of this flap was questioned due to the previous history of pelvic fracture.

Treatment

Routine castration was performed. The perineal space was subsequently explored and hernia contents (prostate gland and periprostatic fat) were identified and reduced. Remnants of the sacrococcygeus and levator ani muscles were identified, along with the external anal sphincter and the sacrotuberous ligament. The internal obturator muscle was fibrotic and atrophied. Therefore, the semitendinosus muscle was chosen as an alternative muscle flap for reconstruction of the perineal diaphragm.

The muscle was approached through an extended incision along the caudal aspect of the thigh (Figure 14.38). The semitendinosus muscle has codominant vascular pedicles, one located proximally and one distally. The muscle will survive on either pedicle. The muscle was dissected, the distal vascular pedicle was ligated and transected, and the proximal vascular pedicle was identified and preserved (Figure 14.39). The proximal pedicle was protected and the origin of the muscle was transected to facilitate rotation of the muscle around the vascular pedicle (Figure 14.40). It is important to protect the pedicle from tension, kinking or compression during subsequent manipulation of the flap.

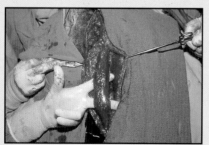

Figure 14.38

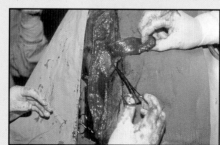

Figure 14.39

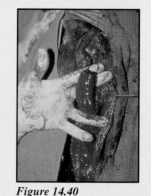

Figure 14.40

CASE SEVEN *continues* ▶

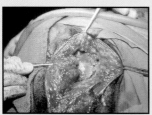

Figure 14.41

Dissection was continued ventral to the ischial arch and into the obturator foramen. The semitendinosus muscle flap was then rotated 180 degrees, and the distal aspect of the muscle was advanced ventral to the ischial arch and through the obturator foramen. The resulting position of the flap was in an ideal location for repair of the perineal diaphragm (Figure 14.41). Margins of the muscle flap were sutured to the external anal sphincter, remnants of the levator ani and coccygeus muscles, and the sacrotuberous ligament. The donor site was closed routinely and dead space was managed using a passive latex (Penrose) drain for 3 days (Figure 14.42).

Outcome

Subsequent healing, limb use and pelvic function was uncompromised.

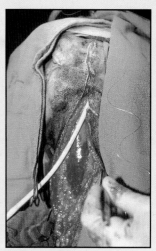

Figure 14.42

CASE EIGHT: Four-year-old spayed female Bull Terrier with a full thickness burn

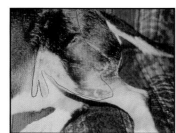

Figure 14.43

History

The bitch was presented to the referring veterinary surgeon acutely, following a thermal injury. She had been trapped beneath the hot exhaust manifold of a car for several minutes. A small full thickness burn was present over the craniolateral aspect of the left tibia and moderate cutaneous oedema was present throughout the left flank (Figure 14.43). No other injuries were present.

Initial treatment

Acute treatment included provision of analgesia using both opioids and NSAIDs. Cold compresses were used locally for an analgesic effect, as well as to help limit progressive tissue injury. Hair was clipped from the region to allow identification and debridement of necrotic tissue. Progressive necrosis resulted in the formation of two large open wounds involving the left flank and lateral thigh. Closure of the flank wound using undermining of local tissues and mesh expansion was attempted (Figure 14.44). The second wound overlying the left thigh remained open.

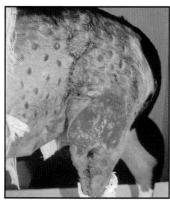

Figure 14.44

Further wound assessment

Tension on wound margins dramatically increases the risk of incisional dehiscence. In this dog, the negative effect of tension was compounded by the location of the wound in the flank fold, an area subjected to excessive motion. Ultimately, this combination of factors led to incisional dehiscence. The bitch was referred for a second opinion 2 weeks later.

Three open wounds were identified: one involving the left flank fold; the second overlying the left thigh; and a third, smaller wound over the craniolateral aspect of the left tibia (Figure 14.45). Mature, but relatively inactive, granulation tissue was present in all wounds. This was visually apparent by the glistening fibrous appearance of the wound bed.

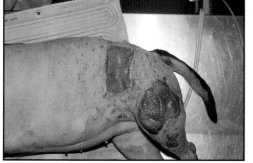

Figure 14.45

CASE EIGHT continues ▶

Management options

Each wound was addressed separately in considering reconstructive options. The flank fold is subject to a great deal of movement; therefore, reconstruction of this area requires the transposition of 'new' tissue into the wound bed. Well vascularized extremity wounds can be reconstructed using many methods. Skin grafts were chosen in this case because of the lateral location of the wounds.

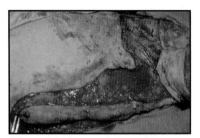

Figure 14.46

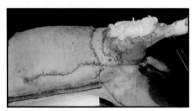

Figure 14.47

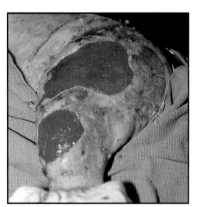

Figure 14.48

Treatment

A caudal superficial epigastric axial pattern skin flap, formed by the caudal mammary glands and dependent upon the caudal superficial epigastric artery and vein which exit the external inguinal ring, was chosen. This flap was easily dissected and transposed into the region of the flank fold (Figure 14.46). Because of the potential for vascular injury during previous tissue undermining and mesh expansion, the integrity of the vascular pedicle was substantiated using a Doppler flow probe prior to surgery. The flap donor site was closed primarily and the flap transposed on to the recipient wound bed (Figure 14.47).

The extremity wounds in this dog were not suitable for immediate reconstruction using skin grafts because of the uneven contour and fibrous nature of the granulation tissue. Superficial debridement of both limb wounds was performed, and the wounds were subsequently bandaged using a bolus tie-over dressing with a petrolatum gauze contact layer. Bandages were changed every other day.

Further assessment of extremity wounds

A well vascularized active granulation bed was established within 5 days of debridement (Figure 14.48). The surface of the wound bed was uniform and the wound was free of necrosis, infection and wound exudation. Application of full thickness skin grafts could be safely considered at this time.

Treatment of extremity wounds

Meshed full thickness skin grafts were harvested from the lateral thorax and stabilized over the wound beds using skin staples (Figure 14.49). Full thickness skin grafts are generally preferred over split thickness grafts since all adnexal structures are transferred with the graft. The mesh incisions allow escape of wound fluid into an overlying absorptive bandage.

The limb required bandaging to limit motion and prevent shear stresses on the graft during the process of revascularization. Bandages were changed after 24 hours and subsequently at 3-day intervals, with complete removal after 14 days.

Outcome

Graft survival was 100% (Figure 14.50).

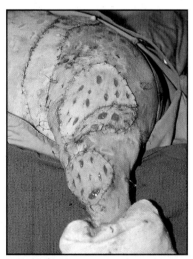

Figure 14.49

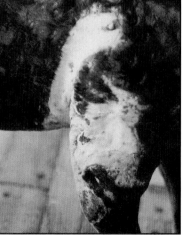

Figure 14.50

CASE NINE: 2-year-old castrated male Domestic Shorthair with hindlimb contracture following degloving injuries

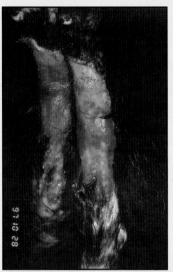

Figure 14.51

History

This cat had had bilateral hindlimb degloving injuries of 3 months duration; the wounds had been debrided and dressed at regular intervals in that period. At presentation, both hindlimbs showed severe contracture and muscle atrophy and the granulation tissue present was chronic with little vascular potential (Figure 14.51). The patient showed severe difficulty in moving his hindlimbs. The cat was tested and found to be negative for both FeLV and FIV; the test was carried out as both viruses have been associated with poor wound healing.

Management options

The main concern was hindlimb function. In order to attempt relatively rapid resolution of the injury, it was thought that excision of the chronic granulation tissue followed by application of a caudal superficial epigastric flap could be used. It was decided that both limbs should not be recontructed simultaneously and a staged procedure was planned.

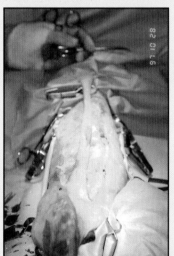

Figure 14.52

Treatment

En bloc debridement of the right limb's granulation bed was carried out down to healthy fascia. A caudal superficial epigastric flap was raised, with its distal extremity at the second mammary gland (Figure 14.52). The flap was rotated into the defect via a bridging incision (Figure 14.53). The wound edges were sutured with simple interrupted sutures of

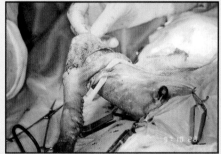

Figure 14.53

2 metric monofilament nylon; no sutures were placed in the body of the flap. The donor site was closed routinely, though it was found to be under some tension. Tension relief was managed by undermining and placement of subcuticular as well as dermal sutures. A Penrose drain was placed for 3 days.

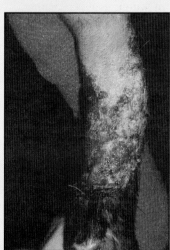

Figure 14.54

Postoperative assessment and further treatment

The flap healed well, though the distal extremity showed some evidence of superficial necrosis (Figure 14.54); this was confined to the most superficial layers and did not affect the final appearance. The donor site dehisced (Figure 14.55) and required management as an open wound, with hydrogel dressings over 7 days until satisfactory closure was achieved.

The problem with the donor site led to a reassessment of the plan for the left leg and it was decided to amputate this limb.

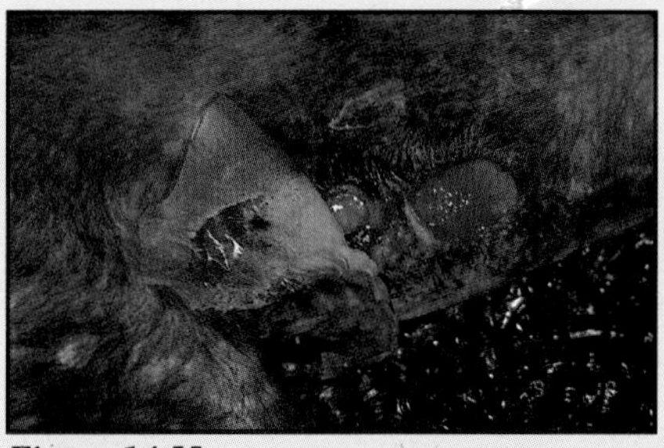

Outcome

The patient made an excellent recovery and is fully mobile 2 years after the surgery.

Figure 14.55

CASE TEN: 5-year-old female Irish Wolfhound with a chronic non-healing elbow wound

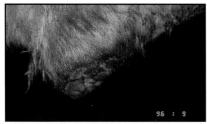

Figure 14.56

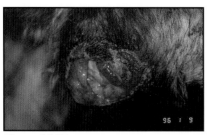

Figure 14.57

History

The bitch was presented with a 12-month history of a non-healing wound over the 'point' of the right elbow (Figures 14.56 and 14.57*)*. About a year earlier she had undergone surgery to excise a hygroma.

Assessment and management options

Swab cultures and biopsy samples revealed no evidence of bacterial infection or neoplasia. Radiographs of the elbow showed no radiographic bony changes.

The problem with excising such a lesion is that any subsequent reconstruction lies over the point of the elbow and will be readily traumatized; dehiscence is a potential problem. Options for managing this case following *en bloc* debridement included: a thoracodorsal artery flap; a transposition flap from the thoracic wall; and the use of multiple releasing incisions. It was decided to use a bipedicled advancement flap. This was to ensure that all suture lines were away from the point of the ulna.

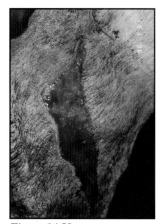

Figure 14.58

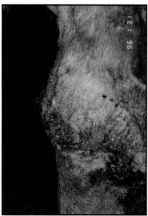

Figure 14.59

Treatment

Following *en bloc* debridement, a releasing incision was made on the medial aspect. The skin of the flap was undermined as deeply as possible to minimize vascular embarrassment. No sutures were placed in the body of the flap and the flap was sutured to the lateral margin of the wound with simple interrupted sutures of 3 metric monofilament nylon. The medial releasing incision was allowed to heal by second intention (Figure 14.58). No dressing was applied to the wounds; this was in order to minimize pressure and potential vascular compromise to the flap.

Outcome

The wound healed with no complications. Although following contraction of the open medial wound the lateral incision had been pulled to the caudal aspect of the elbow (Figure 14.59), no dehiscence occurred.

Index